RED LIGHT, GREEN LIGHT, EAT RIGHT

RED LIGHT, GREEN LIGHT, EAT RIGHT

The Food Solution
That Lets Kids Be Kids

JOANNA DOLGOFF, MD

RODALE

Rodale books may be purchased for business or promotional use or for special sales. For information, please write to: Special Markets Department, Rodale Inc., 733 Third Avenue, New York, NY 10017.

Printed in the United States of America

Rodale Inc. makes every effort to use acid-free ⊗, recycled paper ♺.

Book design by Christina Gaugler

Illustrations by Chris Davidson

Photos on pages 47, 71, 94 (carrots), 151, 153, 154, 155, 188 © Tom MacDonald/Rodale Images. Photos on pages 94 (pear) and 149 © GettyImages/Photodisc. Popcorn photo on page 96 © Thom O'Connor. Almond photo on page 96 © iStockphoto. All others © Mitch Mandel/Rodale Images.

Library of Congress Cataloging-in-Publication Data

Dolgoff, Joanna.
   Red light, green light, eat right : the food solution that lets kids be kids / Joanna Dolgoff.
       p.   cm.
   Includes bibliographical references and index.
   ISBN-13 978–1–60529–484–1 pbk.
    1. Children—Nutrition.   I. Title.
RJ206.D65   2010
613.2083—dc22   2009042728

Distributed to the trade by Macmillan

2   4   6   8   10   9   7   5   3   1   paperback

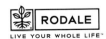

We inspire and enable people to improve their lives and the world around them

For more of our products visit **rodalestore.com** or call 800-848-4735

To my parents, husband, and children for their never-ending love and support.

Without you, none of this would be possible.

Contents

Acknowledgments

● ● ●

I want to thank everybody who helped make this book a reality. My grandpa Marty encouraged me to leave my stable job and take a risk, and to my surprise, my entire family was behind me! I am not sure if I would have had the courage without the support of my parents. Mom and Dad, thank you for making sure I followed my dreams and for reassuring me that you would always be there for me. I never would have been able to do this without you. I would like to thank my in-laws for their love and for always lending a helping hand with the kids. Aunt Robin, you were such a great role model and a true inspiration to me. Jonathan, you have been there for me from the beginning. You are not only my brother, but my friend (and travel agent and maid of honor!). Jason,

thanks for teaching me about business plans and budgets. I shudder to think of what would have happened if you hadn't sat me down and made me focus on the numbers! Amy and Mindy, you are true sisters to me and I love you both. I send my love to my entire family: Grandpa Howie and Anne, Uncle Randy and Aunt Wendy, Aunt Robin and Uncle Robert, Aunt Lisa and Uncle Allen, Aileen and Stuart, and all my incredible cousins. I would like to thank my friends, Dara, Brian, Cynthia, Craig, Patty, Lisa, Scott, Ali, Adam, Shana, and Kara, for spending hours listening to me stress and helping me cope. I am so lucky to have such great friends. Doug, I knew you were my soul mate immediately, despite the fact that you kept swimming away from me. I love you so much. There is nobody else I would rather have by my side, sharing my life. Thanks for your love and support. Zachary and Danielle, I never knew I could feel love so deeply. You make me happier than I ever thought possible. I am really proud of you both.

And to my amazing team . . . Cynthia (aka Cuz, aka Lawyer Extraordinaire), it has been so great working with you that I have to mention you twice! I have loved spending time with you and watching you in action. RoseMarie, you are the best publicist ever. Thanks for taking a chance on me. You were with me from the beginning and I owe so much of my success to you. Dave, Carrie, and TheKBuzz, you helped me turn my idea into a business and taught me the art and importance of social media. Thanks for all your guidance. Celeste, I am so lucky to have found you. You are so

much more than a literary agent! Thank you for putting in all the extra hours and guiding me through this process. Julie, my editor at Rodale, thanks for putting your faith in me and helping me get my program out there. Maggie, I have so enjoyed working with you. Thanks for making this so much fun. Thanks to Alin for his super work on our Web site.

Lori, thank you for all of your hard work and dedication. You are so smart and knowledgeable and you make coming to work fun. I would like to particularly thank you for joining me on all those frozen yogurt runs! I am glad to have you by my side.

But most of all, thanks to the many wonderful patients and parents I have worked with throughout the years. I am thrilled to have been part of your lives and your families. You make my work so meaningful.

Introduction

● ● ●

No parent wants his or her child to be overweight or unhealthy. And if your child is overweight, it can be a scary, frustrating challenge. Along with the serious health issues that accompany excess weight, kids also face emotional, social, and psychological struggles. Overweight kids sometimes suffer from teasing or rejection from classmates, which may cause them to withdraw from typical childhood social experiences such as making new friends, trying out for sports, going to camp, or attending birthday parties. Sometimes even teachers can be biased. No child should have to suffer through the physical or emotional torment of being overweight.

It's no secret that we're in the midst of an obesity epidemic, and kids are tipping the scales just like their parents. One out of every three American children is overweight, and doctors are seeing dangerously obese children as young as age 2. Obesity rates among US children have doubled in the past 20 years. Physicians and public health officials are duly concerned about this worsening problem. And apparently you are, too, or you wouldn't have picked up this book. If you're anxious about whether your child is eating healthfully or is gaining excess weight, you've chosen the right resource. I created *Red Light, Green Light, Eat Right* to help parents and kids learn that optimal health and weight loss can be achieved and maintained *not by restricting food groups or counting calories* but by learning how to eat nutritious foods—and having fun!

Red Light, Green Light, Eat Right is a family nutrition

plan based on the colors of the traffic light: **Green Light** (Go!), **Yellow Light** (Slow!), and **Red Light** (Uh-Oh!). I have color coded more than a thousand foods and determined appropriate serving sizes using this traffic light system. This program is the only standardized weight-loss program for children and teens designed by a physician, so you know it's safe. It's also fun and easy for kids to follow.

Red Light, Green Light, Eat Right encourages the whole family to eat right and exercise more. Overweight family members will follow a program tailored to their weight-loss goals, while healthy-weight family members will follow a program designed for weight maintenance. The end result? Everybody is eating better, together!

So Mom and Dad, even if you don't have a weight problem, you'll benefit from this program. You will eat better and have more energy. And when you participate in the program, you'll have firsthand knowledge of what your kids are experiencing—you'll be excited about it, and you won't feel hypocritical. And your kids will see that the whole family is getting healthy!

I'm sure you're probably wondering if *Red Light, Green Light, Eat Right* will really work for your family. That's understandable. After all, there are so many diets out there, and you may have tried some that just didn't work for you or your kids. Let me reassure you with an encouraging statistic: Because it's fun and

easy to follow, the *Red Light, Green Light, Eat Right* program has a 96 percent success rate. Kids lose weight, get healthier, and don't feel deprived. If you've picked up this book, you've already taken an important first step. Helping your children lose weight is about the smartest move you can make and is a real investment in their future.

Allow me to take a moment here to introduce myself. I am a pediatrician—a doctor who treats infants, children, and teens. I went to Princeton University, majored in molecular biology, and loved every minute of my studies. I also taught exercise classes as a fitness instructor in my spare time. From there, I went on to the New York University School of Medicine, followed by pediatric residency training at Columbia Presbyterian's Children's Hospital of New York. I immediately felt at home in pediatrics. I love working with kids of all ages, and the joy of taking care of children solidified my decision to become a pediatrician. Eventually, I became a general pediatrics practitioner and worked in a private practice for several years.

Although I loved being a pediatrician, I was frustrated by one aspect of it: There were so many overweight kids and not enough time to help them. Most kids generally visited the office because they were sick—they had the chickenpox or the flu, or they needed vaccinations. And even when they visited for other reasons, there just wasn't enough time to have an in-depth conversation with these kids and their parents about the importance of weight management for overall health. I felt helpless about this situation, yet I was determined to do something about it. So I started to intensively research the subject of pediatric weight loss. In doing so, I found that there are two basic types of diets: calorie-restricted diets, in which you eat whatever you want as long as it is within a certain calorie budget; and eating plans that limit unhealthy nutrients or even entire food groups but don't limit calories. Although both types of diets have their merits, neither has really been successful. I wanted to develop a program that combined the best of these two approaches, in which calorie intake was controlled *and* healthier foods were chosen. But the real key was that it had to be designed in a way that a 6-year-old could understand, realistically follow, get needed nutrients, and actually enjoy. What I ultimately created was *Red Light, Green Light, Eat Right.*

Then I took a professional leap of faith. I quit my stable job as a general pediatrician and decided to specialize in pediatric weight loss. Although a lot of people thought I was crazy, my husband and family were all very supportive. I opened up a pediatric weight-loss practice on Long Island and got my first patient right away. Soon my practice started growing by leaps and bounds.

The decision to specialize in pediatric weight loss was the greatest move I've ever made. I am passionate about helping overweight children. I have personally struggled with weight issues throughout my life, trying both healthy and unhealthy diets. Now I'm doing what I love. I'm helping kids. And I'm helping their parents with a program that is both effective and safe. I get to watch my patients lose weight, try out for sports teams for the first time, enjoy active social lives, become more engaged in their schoolwork, and feel better about themselves. And I'm the beneficiary of lots of hugs, handwritten thank-you cards, carefully colored pictures, and inspiring before-and-after photographs.

When overweight kids come to see me, I screen them for medical causes of weight gain and look for subtle signs of medical problems stemming from their weight. I see firsthand the ill effects that excess weight, obesity, and poor diet have on our kids. The health risks are staggering: Diabetes, high blood pressure, and heart disease are just a few of the chronic, life-threatening illnesses faced by today's generation of kids—diseases that were previously limited to adults. It's been documented that kids as young as 5 are being diagnosed with clogged arteries! Even orthopedic problems, resulting from excessive weight on young developing bones, have increased.

In my practice, I see a lot of *acanthosis nigricans.* That's a mouthful, but it refers to a thickening and darkening of the skin around the back of the neck. It's a sign of prediabetes, meaning that the child's body isn't processing insulin normally. If that child doesn't lose weight, he or she will likely develop full-blown type 2 diabetes. Once known as adult-onset diabetes, type 2 diabetes puts kids at risk for very adult ailments, including blindness, nerve damage, kidney failure, and cardiovascular disease. While adults with type 2 diabetes may suffer from these conditions in their sixties or seventies, children with type 2 diabetes will suffer from them in their twenties and thirties! The medical community has suggested that we will soon see more young adults face heart attacks and strokes due to weight-related illnesses. According to a study published in the *Journal of Pediatrics* in 2007, obese kids and teens are more likely to have risk factors associated with cardiovascular disease (such as high blood pressure, high cholesterol, and type 2 diabetes) than are other children and adolescents. In this particular study, which looked at 5- to 17-year-olds, 70 percent of obese children had at least one cardiovascular risk factor, while 39 percent of obese children had two or more cardiovascular risk factors.[1] The childhood obesity epidemic is a ticking time bomb: A 2005 *New England Journal of Medicine* article predicted that because of obesity's negative impact on longevity, the present generation of children and teens may be the first in US history to experience shorter life spans than their parents.[2]

The key to reversing this frightening trend? Parents! Nobody has more influence over your child's health and choices than you do. You are a role model for your children; there's no way around it. The best way to help your child lose weight is to emphasize healthy habits at home.

Even so, a lot of parents I talk to think that "baby fat" will melt away as their kids get older. It won't. The evidence overwhelmingly shows that heavy kids become heavy adults, with higher risks for health problems. In fact, 75 percent of children who are overweight between the ages of 12 and 18 remain obese as adults. And half of overweight children ages 6 to 11 become obese adults. Further, if kids are overweight before 8, they are more likely to be severely overweight as adults.[3]

It's so much easier for kids to lose weight and keep it off if they do so before they enter puberty, that growing-up time of life when hormones start to surge. Boys and girls both bulk up around puberty, with girls gaining more of the weight as fat and boys adding it as muscle. Puberty pounds are tough to budge. There are also changes in children's brains at puberty that control appetite and make them hungrier. And when the teenage years hit, the body establishes a "weight set point," the range of weight the body naturally settles into—and hangs on to. When a teen's weight dips even a little below the set point, the body works to get back to that original set point by lowering metabolism and increasing hunger. This is why most people who lose weight wind up gaining it back. But before this set point is determined, a child can lose weight easily and safely because this response hasn't yet kicked in.

So as a parent, it's important to act as soon as possible, while you have the best chance of making an impact. You are likely to have more influence over the behavior of your younger children than that of your teens. By the time kids become teenagers, they often resist help from their parents. It's tougher, though not impossible, to teach teenagers healthy habits, like listening to their bodies, eating when they're hungry, eating appropriate portions, and leaving food on their plate if they are full.

The good news is that even if your child already has any of the health or psychological problems associated with being overweight, losing weight through good nutrition and exercise can reverse them. Just recently, a young patient who was doing poorly in school came in to see me. His parents and teacher were worried that he might have attention deficit disorder (ADD), and they wanted to have him tested. But after I worked with him to change his diet and he began losing weight, they stopped the evaluation for ADD—because he had become an A student! His parents and his teacher attribute his success in the classroom to the healthy changes he made through following this program.

When you take the important step of addressing your child's weight problem, it's crucial to think of your child's weight as a *family* issue and come together as a family to focus on healthy eating—not on looks, clothing sizes, or "fat" or "thin." Any family can do this, even if one child is overweight and another is not. Healthy eating is for everyone. I'll be the first to admit that getting a family to make healthy choices can be a challenge at times. Not long ago, I went with my husband, Doug, and my two children, Danielle, 4, and Zachary, 7, to a restaurant for dinner. I ordered open-faced whole wheat grilled cheese sandwiches—no butter, no oil—for the kids, with sliced cucumbers on the side. I ordered a large salad for myself. To my dismay, my husband ordered a bacon cheeseburger with large fries! Kids watch everything a parent does. Everyone in the family has to be on board and committed to making healthy changes for the good of the family. Change your own ways, and your kids will change theirs.

Red Light, Green Light, Eat Right will help you encourage nutritious eating habits and regular exercise as a family. I'll give you the tools and information you need to teach your kids—and indeed your whole family—about food, nutrition, and exercise in a fun, meaningful way and to empower everyone to make healthy choices. My hope is that your kids will learn to enjoy a variety of foods, find fun in physical activity, and come to love and appreciate their developing bodies. Here's how this book will help you every step of the way.

● **Lose weight with the power of play!** Based on their age, gender, and goals, kids eat a certain number of **Green Light** foods at each meal and snack. This program accommodates the full spectrum of eaters, from overeaters to picky eaters. Plus, everyone can enjoy the full range of food choices (from chocolate to cheese) and meal options (from home-cooked meals and school lunches to packaged snacks and fast food). A big component of *Red Light, Green Light, Eat Right* is that families with different preferences, lifestyles, and eating styles can realistically share the experience. And there are *no food restrictions*—nothing is off limits!

● **Serve up healthy nutrition.** Are your kids getting the nutrients they need to keep them healthy and alert? That's what most parents want to know, but lately the advice we receive about food seems conflicting and confusing. I'll set the record straight and show you exactly what your child needs to eat each day to nourish his or her growing body.

● **Learn how to make Green Light meals at home.** In the following pages, you'll find more than 50 delicious, easy-to-make recipes for breakfast, lunch, dinner, and snacks. When you cook for your family at home, you know exactly what is going on their plates

and into their bodies—and it's much more budget friendly than buying prepared foods or dining out!

● **Talk to your kids lovingly about weight and health.** You probably have a lot of fears about talking to your kids about weight. The last thing you want to do is make your son or daughter feel self-conscious or ashamed. I'll show you how you can be supportive and helpful without becoming the bad guy or the food police. After all, if you try to restrict too much, your kid's desire for any particular food will only increase.

● **Eat healthfully at restaurants.** According to recent research, kids eat 55 percent more calories while eating out than they do at home. Unfortunately, kids' menus, in general, still consist mainly of low-nutrient, high-calorie foods like pizza, fried chicken nuggets, cheeseburgers, and macaroni and cheese. I'll show you how to navigate around these choices and dine out healthfully at any restaurant.

● **Get your kids moving.** There's no need to sign up your kids for classes at the gym, but it is crucial that they engage in plenty of physical activity. The best way to help them get active is to encourage participation in activities they enjoy doing—things that feel like play, not "exercise." I'll give you some quick, easy, and fun ways to steer your children—and hopefully the whole family—away from the TV and computer and get them up and moving! Remember, the key to success is that Mom and Dad join in, as well.

● **Have a game plan for life.** We know from adult weight-loss studies that the biggest challenge is not losing weight—it's keeping it off. Kids face the same struggle. What you'll learn in this book is how to give your kids lifelong skills to manage their weight and develop healthy attitudes toward food, exercise, and their bodies. That way, eating nutritious foods and exercising will become second nature. All of this helps improve a child's confidence, and that's often the key to maintaining a healthy weight.

There's so much you can do to influence the way your children eat and to lower the chances they will end up with chronic health problems. So gather around the kitchen table . . . and keep reading. You're about to discover that playing with your food has never been so good for you.

1

• • •

COMING TO TERMS: IS YOUR CHILD REALLY OVERWEIGHT?

As a medical doctor and a mom, I'm sometimes surprised when parents fail to recognize that their children have weight problems. "He's big like his dad" and "That's just the way we are in our family" are some of the excuses I've heard from parents whose children have been referred to me. It's natural for parents to see their children as perfect, but you may be overlooking crucial red flags.

Several years ago, a study from Bassett Healthcare Research Institute in Cooperstown, New York, and Columbia University reported that 68 percent of parents of children who were medically classified as obese reported their child's weight as "okay" or "just right." And 8 percent even reported that their child was "underweight"! Clearly, many parents of over-weight kids simply don't realize that their sons and daughters are not healthy.

How can you tell if your child is medically overweight? What does the term *obese* mean when applied to kids? Understanding the facts can help you know when it's time to make healthy changes for your family.

Do a Little Math

As pediatricians, we determine whether a child is overweight or obese through a calculation called body mass index (BMI) percentile. It is a calculation based on height and weight measurements, gender, and age. Ask your child's pediatrician for your child's BMI percentile, or calculate it yourself using the simple formula below. To determine your child's BMI percentile, you must first determine his BMI.

$$BMI = (WEIGHT\ IN\ POUNDS \times 703) \div$$
$$(HEIGHT\ IN\ INCHES \times HEIGHT\ IN\ INCHES)$$

Let's look at an example. Say that Suzy weighs 115 pounds and is 54 inches tall. Here's the math:

$$115\ POUNDS \times 703 = 80,845$$
$$54 \times 54 = 2,916$$
$$80,845 \div 2,916 = 28$$

Suzy would have a BMI of 28.

Once you know your child's BMI, you can determine whether or not she's overweight by consulting a BMI chart. Children's BMI charts are typically color coded by percentiles. Just like the standardized tests your kids take in school, percentile ranking for BMI indicates where your children rank in the spectrum of other kids of the same gender and age. For example, if a child has a BMI in the 70th percentile, 70 percent of the kids of the same gender and age who were measured had a lower BMI. Once you've calculated your child's BMI, write it down. You will use it later to determine which program is appropriate for your child.

Children are classified into four different weight categories based on their BMI. Underweight is less than the 5th percentile; healthy weight is the 5th per-

centile to the 84th percentile; overweight is the 85th percentile to the 94th percentile; and obese is in the 95th to 98th percentile.

The following charts reflect BMI percentiles for boys and girls. To read these charts, look for your child's BMI (vertically) and his age (horizontally). The place where these two points meet is his BMI percentile, shown by the curved lines. If your child falls in the red category, he is considered obese; the yellow category is considered overweight; the green category is normal; and the orange category is underweight.

Boys: BMI for Age Growth Chart

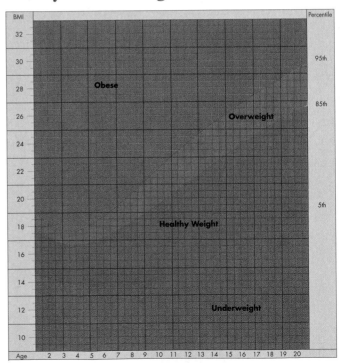

Girls: BMI for Age Growth Chart

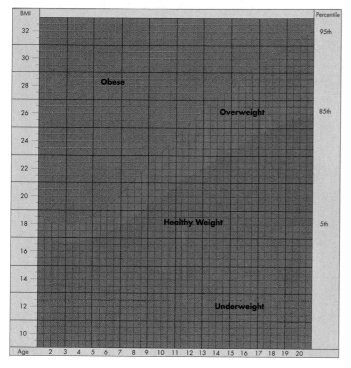

Talking to Your Kids about Weight

If your child has a weight problem, you're probably nervous about broaching the subject with her. Maybe you teeter between making admonitions like "You don't need that dessert" and keeping quiet when she reaches for more food, though your gut tells you otherwise. You might be worried that talking about weight will make her feel overly self-conscious, trigger an obsession with appearance, or even cause an eating disorder or irreparable harm to her self-esteem.

Don't let these worries keep you from initiating the conversation. For starters, most overweight children know they are overweight. Even if you haven't pointed it out, their peers probably have. If you avoid the topic and pretend that everything is fine, your children will learn that their weight is a shameful issue that shouldn't be discussed. They may then try to lose weight on their own, usually by means of ineffective and unsafe measures. So don't wait—begin the conversation. Below are some basic dos and don'ts for talking to kids about weight that I recommend to my patients' nervous parents.

Do:

Use the power of "we." Everyone can benefit from eating a little healthier, so remember to use the word *we* when discussing weight and health. Sit down with your child and discuss your reasons for making changes—say that you want everyone to look and feel their best. For example: "We could all be healthier." "Why don't we try to make some changes together?" "Let's learn how to eat right so we can start getting more active."

Unless you talk in terms of "we," you might send the message that one child has a problem or that he's different from the rest of the family. Using the word *we* sounds less accusatory, more inclusive, and alerts

MEDICAL CONSEQUENCES OF BEING OVERWEIGHT AS A CHILD

- Asthma
- Early puberty
- Gallbladder disease
- Gastrointestinal diseases
- Gout
- Heart disease
- High blood pressure

- High cholesterol
- High triglycerides (fat in the blood)
- Liver disease
- Metabolic syndrome
- Osteoarthritis
- Psychological and social problems

- Sleep apnea (trouble breathing during sleep)
- Shortened life span—even if that person is no longer obese as an adult
- Type 2 diabetes

your child that you and other family members are on the same team. Incidentally, nearly all parents who have participated in *Red Light, Green Light, Eat Right* have lost weight themselves!

Be open—share your own weight struggles. For example, tell your daughter if you experienced a growth spurt in grade school that suddenly made wearing a bathing suit feel awkward. Knowing that you experienced such struggles will help her feel understood and less alone. But avoid negative talk or criticism about your own body—don't say, "Look at Mommy's tummy. She needs to lose weight, too!" When your kids hear you speak negatively about your body, they will become anxious about their own bodies.

Talk to your children about why certain foods are healthier. The word *healthy* can be confusing for children. Instead of just calling a food "healthy"

or labeling foods with value judgments like good or bad, you'll want to explain *why* it's beneficial. Try talking about foods in terms kids can relate to. You can use more scientific explanations for older kids and simplified reasoning for younger kids.

For example, you may tell older kids:

- Spinach contains vitamin E, which helps your skin stay healthy.
- Blueberries are full of antioxidants, which will protect you from disease later in life.
- Eating omega-3 fats in fish and flaxseed allows your brain to perform at its best when you take your math exam.

Younger kids may understand explanations like:

- Eating carrots will help you see better at night when you go trick-or-treating at Halloween.

- Eating broccoli is like eating a tree. You'll grow tall and strong like a tree, too.
- Protein like chicken and fish will build strong muscles and help you do better in soccer.

Explain the relationship between weight and health. Help your child understand that eating unhealthy food and being overweight affect every body system and that there are medical risks associated with being overweight. Modify the discussion based on your child's age. You might simply tell a young child that eating too many Red Light foods can make his heart sick. An older child can handle a more sophisticated explanation of diseases like diabetes and heart disease.

Discuss upcoming food challenges. Families celebrate special occasions with special food. Knowing that a date on the calendar is circled for a party or event where tempting dishes are sure to be served can cause anxiety in a child who is trying to make healthy choices. When possible, ask for the menu in advance so that your child can make informed choices based on the colors of traffic lights. Sit down with your child and map out which foods he plans to eat and which foods he plans to skip. Such planning lets your child enjoy the event without worrying.

Be a shoulder to cry on. Weight loss is not easy, and the day-in, day-out focus and commitment to achieving results can bring up difficult emotions. Encourage your child to express what he's feeling, then listen, listen, listen. Simply allowing children to express their feelings—without immediately trying to fix the problem—will help them feel supported.

Use positive reinforcement. Praise is a powerful tool. Acknowledge every healthy decision, big and small. Praise children when they practice healthy habits. If a child turns down an unhealthy treat, compliment the show of restraint. If a child eats fruit while his friends are eating ice cream, share your pride and celebrate what your family has learned.

Don't:

Sugarcoat by telling heavy children they are not overweight to protect their feelings.

Voice negativity. Never make jokes about a child's weight. If a family member has ever teased you for being heavy, I bet you've never forgotten it. Instead, highlight your child's many attributes—what a good student she is or how well she plays the piano. Positive words can make the difference between a child who addresses her weight problem in a healthful way and one who veers into an unhealthy body image.

Ignore the issue by not talking about it at all. No one wants their kids to grow up feeling badly about themselves. But remember, just because you aren't talking about it doesn't mean your child's peers are not. Silence about weight won't help children or parents. Be loving and supportive when talking about weight.

Offer false platitudes, such as "Don't worry; you'll grow out of it." Remember, overweight kids usually become overweight adults.

Express fatalism. Don't say, "It's in your genes; there's nothing you can do about it." This isn't altogether true. Yes, there are obesity genes that make some kids more likely than others to gain weight. But the genes that make people overweight need an environment to express themselves—an environment in which food is plentiful and high in fat, sugar, and calories. And youngsters will gain weight when they continue to camp out in front of the TV or spend hours playing video games. Genes or not, the answer for our children is simple: They must eat better and move their bodies more.

Talk about weight issues in front of others. Keep siblings, friends, and grandparents out of the discussion. It should be a private conversation.

Compare. We love our children because each one of them is like no other in the world. Keep this in mind when talking to your child about food and weight. Don't say things like "If you would just eat like your sister, you would be fine."

Make it about yourself. Never say things like "I was always skinny. It's a shame you didn't get my genes." Be a good role model. Walk, hike, shoot hoops, ride bikes, play tennis, ski, rake leaves, or do an exercise video with your kids.

Be the food police. You can't control every one of your children's food choices. Nor should you. Too much scrutiny will cause your kids to rebel. Give them enough autonomy and responsibility to learn, by trial and error, the difference between an unhealthy food choice and a healthy one. Resist controlling in favor of planning and partnership. Eventually, they will develop the skills to make healthy choices on their own.

Forbid foods. Outlawing any particular food will only heighten your child's desire for it. Whatever drink or snack you ban will be at the top of the menu when your child has the chance to eat outside of your presence; expect to discover candy wrappers in coat pockets or soda stains on school books. Your child will rebel, both psychologically and physiologically, by overeating and sneaking food. It's a recipe for obesity and disordered eating.

Force foods. This tactic will likely cause aversions that can linger into adulthood. Explain why your children should try the healthy food you've provided, and have patience that your dialogue—not power plays at the dinner table—will convince them to eat new foods.

One More BIG Don't:
Don't Put Kids on Popular Diets!

Low fat, low carb, high protein—there's a diet plan of every flavor. If you're one of the millions of Americans who struggles with weight, you've probably tried them all, or put your kids on one of them, likely with little success. Unlike adults, kids are still growing and developing. During this time, they need a variety of healthy foods to keep their bodies developing properly. The parents of my patients often ask me about the safety of popular diets for their children, and here's my take on it.

● **Low-carbohydrate diets.** I particularly dislike the low-carb trend, especially for children. Despite the results of a 2009 study, which suggest that some low-carb diets might be safe and effective for kids, the American Dietetic Association (ADA) still does not endorse this means of weight loss for children. Kids who eat more low-carb foods are often deficient in fruits and vegetables, fiber, and vitamin C and generally have more body fat. Some side effects that may occur are electrolyte imbalances, dehydration, low potassium levels (hypokalemia), constipation due to inadequate fiber intake, and decreased intake of B vitamins. I do not recommend low-carbohydrate diets for children of any age.

Last year, 10-year-old Kelly came to me with her mother, Diana, to talk about how Kelly could successfully lose 20 pounds. As I talked to mother and daughter about my program, Diana stiffened and said she didn't want Kelly eating "all those carbs." Lured by the promise of quick weight loss, Diana was among the millions of people who believed in low-carb dieting to slim down. She had banned bread, pasta, potatoes, cereals, cookies, and other carbs from the household because she had bought into the fallacy that carbohydrates are evil. Kelly and Diana fought daily because Diana wouldn't let her eat carbs.

I calmly explained that low-carb diets exclude an entire category of macronutrients (carbohydrates), and this is dangerous for children, because they need carbs for energy. Low-carb diets are too high in fat for kids and, among other effects, often don't provide the calcium levels children need to build strong bones. These diets are simply not nutritionally sound.

As we talked, Kelly disclosed that she had been secretly binge eating pasta and bread. Wouldn't it be better if she was permitted to eat many kinds of foods in the right portions, I asked, rather than sneaking unhealthy snacks, gaining weight, and battling over food? Diana saw my point and agreed to put Kelly on my program. Today, Kelly is 20 pounds lighter and much happier. There is peace at home now that Diana realizes that her daughter needs to eat a balanced diet.

● **Very low-calorie diets.** Very low-calorie programs that many adults follow can be dangerous for kids! Children are growing and developing and must eat enough calories to support these changes. A very low-calorie diet (usually under 1,000 calories a day) skimps on food and therefore skimps on nutrients kids need. In fact, these diets may stunt a child's growth. Severe cutbacks in calories are appropriate only in rare circumstances, when prescribed by a doctor who specializes in child and teen weight loss. Children on very low-calorie diets must be monitored to make sure the diet supplies the correct balance of protein, carbohydrates, and fat and that adequate growth is occurring for the child's state of development. I also don't endorse feeding kids meal replacement bars or shakes, which is another form of very low-calorie dieting. I believe it's important for children to eat real foods. I never put patients on very low-calorie programs.

● **High-protein diets.** These diets generally work well for healthy adults, but are not a safe option for kids. A child's body cannot store protein; any excess protein is broken down into amino acids and nitrogen. The amino acids are used for energy or converted to fat, and the nitrogen is excreted by the kidneys and liver. High levels of these waste products have been shown to cause kidney injury and can also harm the liver. Children on high-protein diets may suffer from kidney stones and osteoporosis. What's more, high-protein diets limit intake of healthy foods, such as whole grains, fruits, and vegetables. High-protein foods are also usually high in fat and cholesterol, which may increase the risk of heart disease, stroke, and other health problems in kids.

● **Low-fat diets.** Low-fat diets (with less than 20 percent of total calorie intake coming from fat) are appealing to many adults, but they aren't healthy for kids. Fats are essential for children's growing bodies and developing brains. Studies have not been done on very low-fat diets in children because it is clear that children must have sufficient fat in their diets to fuel growth and brain development (which continues throughout childhood).

● **Diet pills.** The use of diet pills, appetite suppressants, and herbal supplements for weight loss is dangerous for both adults and children. Over-the-counter (OTC) diet pills and appetite suppressants may contain large amounts of caffeine. Caffeine can cause abnormally fast heart rates in children. Many OTC weight-loss supplements haven't been approved by the FDA for use in children or adults.

The diet methods listed above not only are unhealthy for children, but also are difficult for children to follow and severely restrict their options. Kids face the added pressure of frequent class activities, parties, and play dates where they have no control over what foods are served. If a child were following a low-carbohydrate diet, he would never be able to enjoy a piece of pizza or a slice of cake. What kind of childhood is that? I believe that all food groups should be enjoyed in moderation and in the correct portion sizes.

Some studies have shown that months after following adult diets, children actually weigh *more* than before they started. So instead of putting your whole family on a grown-up diet trend, now's the time to do something different. *Red Light, Green Light, Eat Right* will work for you and your family because it provides what most diets don't: a fun way to manage weight, learn about nutrition, and get healthy. It's a way of life, too—one that brings about lasting changes in your kids' weight and lets them enjoy an energetic, healthy lifestyle. Best of all, it's a game that the whole family can play . . . so let's start playing!

2

● ● ●

LEARNING THE RULES OF THE ROAD

One day when my daughter, Danielle, was only 3 years old, she looked up from her lunch and asked me how many calories were in her turkey sandwich. I always wanted my children to be aware that some foods were healthy and some were not. But *calories*? She was just a kid!

I took a moment to collect myself. "Honey," I said, "a turkey sandwich on whole wheat bread is a very healthy food." I thought for a moment more. "In fact, it is a Green Light food. Don't worry about calories. Just try to make good choices and eat Green Light foods."

"Okay, Mommy!" she smiled. Simple enough. And so we began using the colors of the traffic light and its familiar messages to make healthier choices. With

this approach, there's no complicated calorie counting. No foods are off-limits. And your child will lose excess weight and get the nutrition she needs!

One example of the plan's success is 8-year-old Sammy, who came to see me with his mom on the advice of their regular pediatrician. Sammy was 98 pounds and medically obese for his age and height. He often refused to go to school because his classmates teased him about his weight. His mother felt that Sammy's eating was out of control, but she didn't know how to help him. I explained the traffic light system to Sammy and his mom and showed them how to tailor the program to his specific needs and goals.

Ten weeks later, he had lost 14½ pounds. While he

was still overweight, Sammy was no longer in the dangerous "obese" category. He had more energy to keep up with his friends at school and was able to join the soccer team. His self-confidence soared, and his classmates stopped teasing him. In less than 3 months, Sammy became a healthier, happier young man. And because he found his game plan easy to follow, enjoyed being on it, and saw results, he stuck with it and today maintains a healthy weight for his height and age.

Red Light, Green Light, Eat Right has also worked wonders for parents with normal-weight children. Melinda and Helen were 6- and 8-year-old cousins who took picky eating to the extreme. Melinda was subsisting on just three foods—Cheerios, plain pasta, and raisins—which offered some fiber but little in the way of calcium, protein, or iron. Helen steadfastly refused to eat anything but American cheese, white bread, and potato chips. She easily got full, but she was starving for nutrients. Both girls were skinny, but they weren't healthy. Melinda could not expect to grow normally without eating protein, and Helen was on a clear path to weight gain and high cholesterol. It was time for some serious problem solving. I showed their parents how to use the traffic light system for weight maintenance, and both girls learned to eat—and enjoy—a healthy diet that supplies the nutrients they need to grow strong bodies.

As you can see, Sammy, Helen, and Melinda faced different challenges when it came to eating and nutrition—but *Red Light, Green Light, Eat Right* helped all of them get healthy. And it can do the same for your children. Here's how it works.

Green Light Foods (GO!)

In general, **Green Light** foods are high in nutrient value and lower in calories and fat. Most Green Light foods contain protein, fiber, and other nutrients—and thus are very healthy. The actual color of a food does not always match the traffic light color.

Lean proteins such as fish, skinless chicken, and fat-free hot dogs count as Green Light foods. So do starches like potatoes, brown rice, whole wheat bread, and many types of cereals. Fat-free milk is a Green Light food, too.

While this eating plan has been created with children's nutritional needs in mind, I've also included what I call "junky" Green Light foods. Sometimes when our kids beg to try new snacks—or when soccer practice, dance rehearsal, and work schedules collide—packaged foods such as 100-calorie packs, baked potato chips, and reduced-fat Chips Ahoy! cookies are convenient solutions. They may not provide lots of nutrition, but in the right portions, they're low in calories and will keep your kids from feeling deprived of the foods they want to eat. You'll be pleasantly surprised when you see the many Green Light foods your kids are able to choose from. And the best way for them to get all of the vitamins, minerals, and other nutrients they need each day is to eat a variety of foods.

In the food database located in this book's Appendix, I've placed asterisks next to the most nutritious options. Whenever possible, you and your child will want to select as many of these healthy Green Light foods as possible, like fat-free or low-fat yogurt; whole grain breads and cereals; and lean proteins like fish, chicken, and lean beef. Not only are these foods lower in calories, most are very satisfying. Your children will feel fuller when they choose to eat these wholesome Green Light foods.

Yellow Light Foods (SLOW!)

Yellow Light foods are moderately high in calories and slightly higher in fat than Green Light foods. Yellow Light foods still provide healthy nutrition, but they should be eaten in moderation. Examples of Yellow Light foods include olive oil, granola bars, dark chocolate, and ice cream. These foods can be included in a child's daily diet if eaten in the right portions.

For Yellow Light protein, you can choose from options like ground beef, chicken nuggets, and pork chops. There are also main dishes kids love, like macaroni and cheese and spaghetti and meatballs. Kids love cereals, too, and there are more than 20 Yellow Light cereals on the plan.

Red Light Foods (UH-OH!)

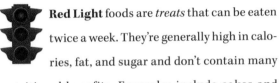

Red Light foods are *treats* that can be eaten twice a week. They're generally high in calories, fat, and sugar and don't contain many nutritional benefits. Examples include cakes and pies, fried chicken, and fried mozzarella.

Combination Foods

Many foods on this plan are "combination" foods. They rate as **Green Light** + **Yellow Light** foods, **Yellow Light** + **Red Light** foods, or **Green Light** + **Red Light** foods because they're a mixture of higher- and lower-calorie foods. Enchiladas, for example, are a **Green Light** + **Yellow Light** food. When your child eats them, he uses both a **Green Light** *and* a **Yellow Light** for that meal. Many fast foods fit into the **Yellow Light** + **Red Light** or **Green Light** + **Red Light** categories. Including combination foods as part of the plan gives you and your family lots of flexibility and choices, especially when eating out.

Free Fuel

Free Fuel foods are unlimited and do not count as traffic lights of any color. All fresh or frozen fruits and vegetables are Free Fuel—except for potatoes, corn, some beans, and avocados, which are each one Green Light per serving. These Free Fuel foods are high in fiber, which promotes satiety, or the feeling of fullness, so your child is less likely to overindulge in them. Dried fruits, such as raisins, are *not* Free Fuel. They can be included in a healthy diet but must be accounted for. Only *fresh or frozen* fruits and vegetables are Free Fuel.

Fat-free cheese is another option for Free Fuel and is also a good source of calcium. Cheese must be 100 percent fat free to count as Free Fuel. Low-fat, reduced-fat, part-skim, and 2 percent cheeses are not Free Fuel. They can still be included in your child's diet, but each serving must be counted as a Green Light (see "Cheese" in the Appendix at the back of the book). Also note that not all fat-free dairy products are Free Fuel. Foods like fat-free milk and fat-free yogurt, while nutritious, are Green Lights, not Free Fuel.

Choose from More Than 1,000 Foods!

At the back of this book you'll find an index of more than 1,000 foods that have been nutritionally assessed and coded by color along with their appropriate serving size. You and your children can use this database to decide what to eat. Because foods are listed by category, you can quickly find the healthiest version of a food or an ingredient. For example, if you were to look in the "Ice Cream and Toppings" section, you'd find that low-fat frozen yogurt is a **Green Light** food, while chocolate sorbet is a **Yellow Light** food; if you looked under "Meat, Meat Dishes, and Lunch Meats," you'd discover that bologna is a **Yellow Light** food while Canadian-style bacon is a **Green Light** food. And don't forget, the most healthy, nutrient-dense foods are marked with an asterisk. Try to choose these foods for your child as frequently as possible.

The options are endless! At first, expect to refer to the database often, but the longer you incorporate this game plan into your family's life, the less you'll need to consult it. Eating foods based on traffic light colors, and building meals around them, will become second nature to you and everyone else in your family.

It's time to start your engines and get on the road to a healthier life for your whole family. Here are the *Red Light, Green Light, Eat Right* rules of the road.

Mind the Traffic Lights!

Now that you understand how foods are categorized into Red, Yellow, and Green Lights, talk to your kids about what kinds of foods are what kinds of colors. My advice is to sit down with your children and let them know that you want to start this program to help everyone in the family get healthier. Do this at a neutral time when they're not hungry, like after a meal. You can start by showing them the database of Green Light, Yellow Light, and Red Light foods in the Appendix and the photos of the delicious recipes in this book. Highlight the foods your children like. Get excited about the options. Talk about how many choices there are and how yummy the foods are. Show enthusiasm!

If your child is younger, perhaps you can use a recent meal as an example—explain which lights were represented. Let them know that Green Light foods should always be their first choice, Yellow Light foods represent caution and should be eaten in moderation, and Red Light foods are occasional treats. Explain that they must stop and really think about whether or not they want to eat a Red Light food before choosing it. Help them understand that treats are less special when you can have them every day.

As they become more familiar with the plan, take your children grocery shopping and ask them to point out which foods are Green Lights, Yellow Lights, or Red Lights. Once you're home, you can make a game with green, yellow, and red stickers or markers: Let your kids apply stickers or draw dots on corresponding foods in the pantry and fridge. This will reinforce their new learning and make it easy for them to choose healthy meals and snacks on the go.

Another fun activity is to draw a daily calendar on a white poster board or even a simple sheet of paper and have your kids fill in their lights for each day as colored dots. Then, after they eat every meal and snack, they can stick on a corresponding sticker as they use up their lights. Not only does this help them keep track of their lights, it also turns nutrition into a game they'll enjoy.

Find Your Game Plan for Weight Loss

If your child needs to lose weight, Road Rule 2 will help you determine the appropriate plan. If your child does not need to lose weight, you may skip to Road Rule 3.

Children should eat a specified number of Green Light foods at each meal and snack, based on their age, gender, and BMI. You'll find several different game plans on the following pages. Look through these options and select the plan that fits your child's needs. You'll need to refer to your child's BMI measurement that you calculated in Chapter 1.

WEIGHT LOSS GAME PLANS

Girls 4–6 (BMI 17.4–24); Girls 7–8 (BMI 18–24); Girls 9–10 (BMI 20–26.5); Boys 4–6 (BMI 17.1–21); and Boys 7–8 (BMI 17.6–22.5)				
BREAKFAST	MORNING SNACK	LUNCH	AFTERNOON SNACK	DINNER
●●	●	●●●	●	●●●

Girls 4–6 (BMI 24.1–30); Girls 7–8 (BMI 24.1–30.5); Girls 9–10 (BMI 26.6–32); Girls 11–12 (BMI 21.5–29); Girls 13–14 (BMI 23.1–31.5); Girls 15–16 (BMI 24.6–33.5); Girls 17–18 (BMI 25.6–35); Girls 19 and Older, including Moms (BMI 26.6–36); Boys 4–6 (BMI 21.1–26); Boys 7–8 (BMI 22.6–28.5); and Boys 9 (BMI 19.1–25)				
BREAKFAST	MORNING SNACK	LUNCH	AFTERNOON SNACK	DINNER
●●	●	●●●	●●	●●

Girls 4–6 (BMI >30); Girls 7–8 (BMI >30.5); Girls 9–10 (BMI >32); Girls 11–12 (BMI 29.1–33.5); Girls 13–14 (BMI 31.6–35); Girls 15–16 (BMI 33.6–36); Girls 17–18 (BMI 35.1–37); Girls 19 and Older, including Moms (BMI 36.1–38); Boys 4–6 (BMI >26); Boys 7–8 (BMI >28.5); Boys 9 (BMI 25.1–31); and Boys 10–11 (BMI 20.1–26.5)				
BREAKFAST	MORNING SNACK	LUNCH	AFTERNOON SNACK	DINNER
●●	●	●●●	●●	●●●●

Girls 11–12 (BMI >33.5); Girls 13–14 (BMI >35); Girls 15–16 (BMI >36); Girls 17–18 (BMI >37); Girls 19 and Older, including Moms (BMI >38); Boys 9 (BMI >31); and Boys 10–11 (BMI 26.6–32)				
BREAKFAST	MORNING SNACK	LUNCH	AFTERNOON SNACK	DINNER
●●	●	●●●●	●●	●●●●

WEIGHT LOSS GAME PLANS

Boys 10–11 (BMI >32); Boys 12–13 (BMI 21.6–28.5); and Boys 20 and Older, including Dads (BMI 27.1–35.5)

BREAKFAST	MORNING SNACK	LUNCH	AFTERNOON SNACK	DINNER
●●	●●	●●●●	●●	●●●●

Boys 12–13 (BMI 28.6–34.5); Boys 14–15 (BMI 22.1–29.5); Boys 20 and Older, including Dads (BMI 35.6–38.5)

BREAKFAST	MORNING SNACK	LUNCH	AFTERNOON SNACK	DINNER
●●	●●	●●●●	●●	●●●●●

Boys 12–13 (BMI >34.5); Boys 14–15 (BMI 29.6–35.5); and Boys 20 and Older, including Dads (BMI >38.5)

BREAKFAST	MORNING SNACK	LUNCH	AFTERNOON SNACK	DINNER
●●●	●●	●●●●	●●	●●●●●

Boys 14–15 (BMI >35.5) and Boys 16–17 (BMI 24.6–32)

BREAKFAST	MORNING SNACK	LUNCH	AFTERNOON SNACK	DINNER
●●●	●●	●●●●●	●●	●●●●●

Red Light, Green Light, Eat Right

Boys 16–17 (BMI 32.1–36.5) and Boys 18–19 (BMI 26.1–34)				
BREAKFAST	MORNING SNACK	LUNCH	AFTERNOON SNACK	DINNER
● ● ●	● ●	● ● ● ● ●	● ● ●	● ● ● ● ●

Boys 16–17 (BMI >36.5) and Boys 18–19 (BMI 34.1–37.5)				
BREAKFAST	MORNING SNACK	LUNCH	AFTERNOON SNACK	DINNER
● ● ●	● ● ●	● ● ● ● ●	● ● ●	● ● ● ● ●

Boys 18–19 (BMI >37.5)				
BREAKFAST	MORNING SNACK	LUNCH	AFTERNOON SNACK	DINNER
● ● ●	● ● ●	● ● ● ● ●	● ● ● ●	● ● ● ● ●

As you can see, the plans call for three meals and two snacks each day, which means kids will eat about every 3 to 4 hours. Eating throughout the day will rev up their metabolism (the rate at which the body burns calories) and increase the efficiency with which their bodies burn calories.

Your child will lose weight safely and gradually. As pounds melt away, his or her BMI will change. It's important to continue to monitor kids' BMI at least once a month and adjust their game plans accordingly.

Find Your Game Plan for Eating Healthy

Even if your family isn't overweight, they can all benefit from eating more nutritious foods, which will help them to feel their best and avoid health problems. On the following pages, you'll find several game plans for weight maintenance based on age, gender, and BMI.

HEALTHY EATING GAME PLANS

Boys 4–6 (BMI <17) and Girls 4–6 (BMI <17.3)

BREAKFAST	MORNING SNACK	LUNCH	AFTERNOON SNACK	DINNER
●●	●	●●●●	●	●●●●

Boys 7–8 (BMI <17.5); Boys 9–10 (BMI <19); Girls 7–8 (BMI <17.9); Girls 9–10 (BMI <19.9); Girls 11–12 (BMI <21.4); and Girls 17–18 (BMI <25.5)

BREAKFAST	MORNING SNACK	LUNCH	AFTERNOON SNACK	DINNER
●●	●●	●●●	●●	●●●●

Girls 13–14 (BMI <23); Girls 15–16 (BMI <24.5); and Boys 11–12 (BMI <20)

BREAKFAST	MORNING SNACK	LUNCH	AFTERNOON SNACK	DINNER
●●●	●●	●●●	●●	●●●●

Boys 12–13 (BMI <21.5) and Boys 20 and Older, including Dads (BMI <27)

BREAKFAST	MORNING SNACK	LUNCH	AFTERNOON SNACK	DINNER
●●●	●●●	●●●	●●●	●●●●●

Red Light, Green Light, Eat Right

HEALTHY EATING GAME PLANS

Boys 14–15 (BMI <22)				
BREAKFAST	MORNING SNACK	LUNCH	AFTERNOON SNACK	DINNER
● ● ●	● ● ●	● ● ● ● ●	● ● ●	● ● ● ● ●

Boys 16–17 (BMI <24.5)				
BREAKFAST	MORNING SNACK	LUNCH	AFTERNOON SNACK	DINNER
● ● ●	● ● ●	● ● ● ● ●	● ● ● ● ●	● ● ● ● ●

Boys 18–19 (BMI <26)				
BREAKFAST	MORNING SNACK	LUNCH	AFTERNOON SNACK	DINNER
● ● ● ●	● ● ●	● ● ● ● ●	● ● ● ● ●	● ● ● ● ●

Girls 19 and Older, including Moms (BMI <26.5)				
BREAKFAST	MORNING SNACK	LUNCH	AFTERNOON SNACK	DINNER
● ●	● ●	● ● ● ●	● ●	● ● ● ●

Serve This . . . for a Healthy, Balanced Diet

When preparing meals for your family, it's important to pay attention to good nutrition. Make sure your children eat a combination of protein, milk and dairy foods, grains, healthy fats, fruits, and vegetables each day. You'll find recipes and ideas throughout this book to help you create healthy meals and snacks your kids will love. This chart provides a basic overview of foods that should be included in your children's diets.

FOOD GROUP OR NUTRIENT	HEALTHY OPTIONS
Protein	Meat, fish, eggs, poultry, dairy products, and plant foods like nuts and beans
Grains (carbohydrates)	Whole grain cereals, brown or wild rice, whole grain breads, and whole grain crackers
Vegetables	Broccoli, brussels sprouts, cabbage, carrots, cauliflower, cucumbers, green beans, lettuce, onion, pumpkin, spinach, sweet potatoes, and tomatoes
Fruit	Apple, banana, berries, grapes, melon, orange, pear, pineapple, and watermelon
Dairy	Fat-free (skim) milk, low-fat or fat-free yogurt, and low-fat or fat-free cheeses
Fats	Olive oil, nuts, peanut butter, and avocados

ROAD RULE 4

Never Skip Meals or Snacks

This is one of the most common and unfortunate weight-loss mistakes many families make. Although your children may initially consume fewer calories by skipping meals, they will almost certainly become so hungry that they will eat too much at their next meal or snack. In fact, studies show that children who skip meals eat *more* per day than children who eat all their meals.[1] (Incidentally, the same goes for adults, so moms and dads: Eat your breakfast!)

Think of your child's metabolism like a fire. In order for that fire to provide kids with energy, it needs fuel to keep it burning strong throughout the day. Each meal or snack is like a piece of wood that keeps their metabolism raging all day long—and thus burning calories and fat. Skip a meal or snack and the fire dies out!

Use Your Free Fuel

The great thing about Free Fuel is that you and your kids can eat as much of it as you'd like throughout the day without using any of your traffic lights. Free Fuel is nutritious and low in calories and fat. It should be eaten with every meal and snack. *In fact, children must eat a fruit or vegetable with each meal and snack for their game plans to work!* That way, they'll automatically meet their daily requirements for fruit and vegetable servings. Free Fuel encourages kids to make healthy choices when they are hungry. When they fuel up with these "free" sources of vitamins, minerals, calcium, and antioxidants, they're learning healthy habits.

Enjoy Your Pit Stops!

Here's one of the parts of the plan that kids love most: They get to make two weekly pit stops at Red Lights. Yes, it's okay for them to occasionally choose Red Light foods! An eating plan that doesn't incorporate favorite foods is destined to fail because it makes kids feel deprived, which can lead to secret eating, sneaking treats, and other unhealthy habits. Allowing your kids to indulge in Red Light foods in moderation will help them *lose*, not gain, weight over the long haul and encourages a healthy relationship with food. Kids need to learn how to enjoy treats and indulgences without going overboard. In short: Kids should be allowed to be kids! I can't imagine a childhood that doesn't include an ice-cream cone at the boardwalk or one of Grandma's special cookies.

Just remember: only two Red Light foods a week. However, if your child goes over that limit—or "runs a red light"—don't be too hard on her. I believe in progress, not perfection. Just get your child back on track—which is exactly what one of my patients, Marcy, did after a birthday party.

When Marcy came into my office, she was extremely upset and practically in tears. She had been following her game plan perfectly for a month and had already lost an incredible 5 pounds. But she went to a birthday party and felt that she blew it. Although she was out of Red Light foods for the week, she ate two large cookies. That week, she didn't lose any weight.

"What did you do the day after the party?" I asked.

"I started over and followed the plan," she told me. "Then I'm proud of you!"

She looked at me in surprise. I told her that everybody veers off course now and again. The important part is getting right back on track and moving forward. I told her to look at it as a learning experience. The next time she was going to go to a party, we could come up with a game plan so she wouldn't run another red light.

Marcy returned to her healthy eating, and she lost 2 more pounds the following week. Nobody plays every game perfectly 100 percent of the time, and it will take your child a little while to get used to the rules of the road. The key is to get her back to her game plan as soon as possible!

ROAD RULE 7

Mix and Match Your Lights

2 Green Lights = 1 Yellow Light
2 Yellow Lights = 1 Red Light

You may have noticed neither the weight-loss nor the healthy-eating game plans include Yellow Lights. If your child wants to eat a Yellow Light food, all he has to do is trade in two Green Light foods. He can also trade in a Red Light food and eat two Yellow Lights instead. Swapping colors helps kids understand the fundamentals of the plan and gives them even more choices. I use this trading technique to teach children a basic principle of healthy eating: If they choose healthier or lower-calorie foods, they get to eat more. Of course, the key to staying full is to choose healthier foods whenever possible.

Let's say one morning your daughter decides she doesn't want her usual two–**Green Light** breakfast: a serving of Cheerios (¾ cup) with fat-free milk (1 cup). She can trade in these two **Green Light**s and eat one **Yellow Light** instead. So instead of cereal with milk she could have a serving of FRENCH TOAST (page 41), a **Yellow Light** food, with sugar-free syrup (**Free Fuel**) and a cup of sliced strawberries (**Free Fuel**). Or she could try the BREAKFAST QUESADILLA (page 38), also a **Yellow Light** food, paired with a banana (**Free Fuel**).

Here's another example. Suppose your son's baseball team is going to Pizza Hut after a big game, and he's decided he wants to use one of his weekly pit stops for the special occasion. Instead of ordering one slice of Meat Lover's Pizza (**Red Light**), he could choose two slices of plain pizza (two **Yellow Lights**). That way he can make the most of his pit stop and feel satisfied with his meal.

Every once in a while, a child looks at me with a sly grin and asks, "So does that mean I can give up all my Greens and just eat Reds?" Luckily, that's impossible to do, since every child—no matter which game plan they're following—gets only two Red Light foods each week!

You Can Turn Calories into Colors

The foods listed in the Appendix have been coded by traffic light color based on serving size, calories, fat, protein, and fiber. However, in a pinch, as long as you know a food's calorie content, you can determine the color value for your child. Here is the conversion chart.

CALORIES	COLOR
0–100	**Green**
101–200	**Yellow**
201–300	**Yellow + Green**
301–400	**Red**
400 +	**Red** + add one **Green** for every additional 100 calories

Start Your Day with a Clean Slate!

Every single day is a new race day! Stay on track with three meals and two snacks per day. Rearrange color combinations as desired. Have fun with it all. And remember, when players reach the finish line, they have completed the day. *Any unused servings are lost.* This prevents kids from saving up Greens or Yellows to eat the next day or hoarding 5 Reds to eat at the end of the month. Always remind your children that tomorrow is a new day to play. Do-overs are not only allowed, they're mandatory!

Kids Learn to Make Healthy Choices on Their Own

Uniquely, this kid-friendly program empowers your children to make healthier choices for *themselves*—a positive nutrition habit they'll carry throughout their lives. For example, my 7-year-old son Zachary's favorite lunch is an egg salad sandwich. One-half cup of egg salad is a **Red Light** food, and one slice of white bread is a **Green Light** food, which means a typical egg salad sandwich on two pieces of white bread would be **Green Light, Green Light, Red Light** (uh-oh!). But Zachary can easily lower the color value of his egg salad sandwich and make it healthier by making a few minor changes. He makes the egg salad with one egg (**Green Light**) instead of two eggs (**Green Light, Green Light**) and 2 tablespoons of fat-free mayonnaise (**Free Fuel**) instead of regular mayonnaise (**Yellow Light**). Then he places the healthier egg salad on two slices of reduced-calorie, whole wheat bread (**Green Light**). He has successfully changed his

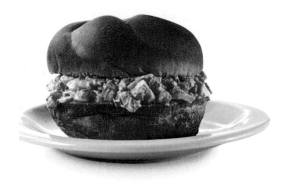

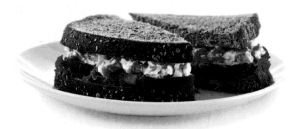

favorite Saturday lunch from **Green Light, Green Light, Red Light** to **Green Light, Green Light.** This means he can use his **Red Light** pit stop for something else later in the week.

There are so many foods, including Free Fuel, that can be interchanged with one another that this substitution strategy can work for almost anything. Most of the time, kids don't even taste the difference. And there is no tricking or deception, no complicated calculations to confuse their food choices. Any meal can be transformed into a healthy meal once your kids understand the colors of the traffic light.

Keep Your Eyes on Portion Size!

My 10-year-old patient Sari was trying to lose weight, without much success. Her mother told me Sari had really changed her eating habits: "We never eat fast food anymore, and we pack her a healthy lunch to take to school each day. Our dinners consist of a healthy protein with a whole grain and vegetables. And she stopped eating dessert after dinner." Sari added, "I even eat salad with low-fat dressing with lunch and dinner. Why am I not losing any weight?"

I had a feeling I knew the answer. Sari and I sat down and reviewed a sample day of her meals and snacks. We went through the food lists and, using measuring cups, estimated her portion sizes. The culprit was as I suspected: portion distortion! Sari was eating the right foods, but she was consuming two to three times the correct portion size. Doubling or tripling portions can turn **Green Lights** into **Yellow Lights** and **Red Lights** because as portions increase, so do calories. Even healthy foods have calories! If children eat too much of anything, they will gain weight. I taught Sari how to use common items familiar to kids to understand portions, and she was able to get her game plan back on track.

USING COMMON ITEMS TO MEASURE FOOD PORTIONS

ITEM	EQUIVALENT MEASUREMENT	FOODS
CELL PHONE OR COMPUTER MOUSE	3 oz	Meat Fish Poultry
BASEBALL	1 c	Rice, pasta Cereal Veggies Chopped fresh fruit or 1 piece of whole fruit
4 MARBLES	1 oz	Hard cheese
1 CHECKER	1 Tbsp	Peanut butter Mayonnaise Low-fat mayonnaise Salad dressing

How can your children practice portion control without becoming hungry? The chart above uses common household items your kids are familiar with to help them estimate appropriate portion sizes for food. Giving them these examples will help them eyeball the right serving without having to measure or weigh food.

Kids' Hunger Scale

What is hunger? Hunger is an important message our bodies send to our brains when they need more nutrients for growth, repair, and energy. Hunger feels like hollowness in the stomach, and sometimes it rumbles and grumbles. Once hunger starts, your child's energy stores are running low. It's difficult for a hungry child to be active, concentrate on activities, or do well on school assignments. And sometimes hunger makes kids irritable or gives them headaches. So it's important to teach children how to recognize hunger and relieve it by eating healthy foods.

The Kids' Hunger Scale on the following page

helps teach children when to eat. If they aren't hungry and they force themselves to eat just because it's lunchtime, for instance, then they won't learn to listen intuitively to what their bodies need. Or if they wait to eat until they get too hungry, they might overindulge, since excessive hunger leads to overeating.

Using the tool below, kids can learn to rate their hunger on a scale from 0 to 4, with 0 being not yet hungry and 4 being ravenous. For younger kids, I relate these numbers to animals—hungry as a bird, hungry as a horse, hungry as a bear, or hungry as a wolf. These descriptions not only help children understand the signals the body sends when they are hungry, but make a game out of it.

KIDS' HUNGER SCALE

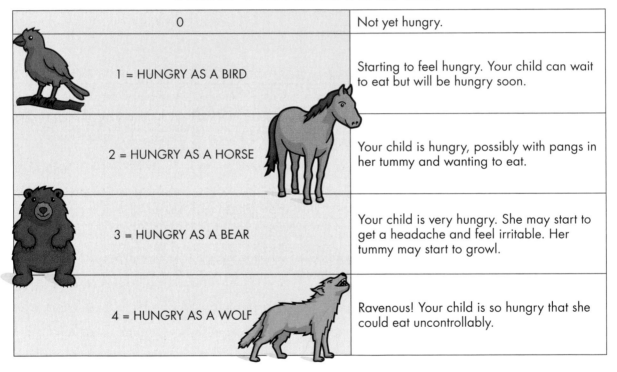

0	Not yet hungry.
1 = HUNGRY AS A BIRD	Starting to feel hungry. Your child can wait to eat but will be hungry soon.
2 = HUNGRY AS A HORSE	Your child is hungry, possibly with pangs in her tummy and wanting to eat.
3 = HUNGRY AS A BEAR	Your child is very hungry. She may start to get a headache and feel irritable. Her tummy may start to growl.
4 = HUNGRY AS A WOLF	Ravenous! Your child is so hungry that she could eat uncontrollably.

The goal is to have kids eat when they get to level 2 (hungry as a horse). Never let your child get to level 4 (hungry as a wolf), or there's the likelihood of overeating or choosing unhealthy foods. At that point, the body just wants to take in as many calories as possible in as short a time as possible and

Red Light, Green Light, Eat Right

craves fat and carbohydrates, often in the form of empty calories. It's not easy to control kids' eating when their blood sugar dips low—they really will eat like wolves!

The Kids' Fullness Gauge

Whereas the Hunger Scale teaches kids when to eat, the Kids' Fullness Gauge (at right) shows them to stop eating when they're full. It uses a representation of a fuel gauge on a car to help kids understand when they've eaten enough.

Explain to your children that their tummies are like the gas tank in the family car. When the fuel gauge on a car indicates that the tank is close to empty, Mommy starts looking for a gas station. The same is true of the body. Kids should avoid running on empty or they'll run out of energy. By thinking of their tummies as a gas tank, they can assess how full they feel. Use the following visual with your children to explain fullness.

- **Empty to ¼ tank:** Low on fuel. Continue to eat. If your child stops eating, he or she will definitely be hungry again soon.
- **½ tank:** Not hungry, but not yet full. If they stop eating, children might get hungry again within the next hour.
- **¾ tank:** Almost a full tank. Your child is begin-

KIDS' FULLNESS GAUGE

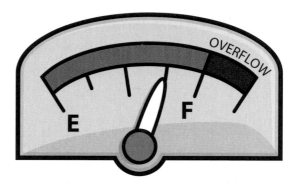

ning to feel comfortable and can go 3 to 5 hours until eating again.
- **Full tank:** The feeling of complete fullness should pass in about 30 minutes.
- **Overflow:** Tank is running over! A child may have eaten too much and feels uncomfortably stuffed.

Ideally, children should be at ¾ tank to full when finishing a meal or snack. You might have everyone pause in the middle of a meal to ask, "How full am I?" If they are still very hungry, they should continue eating. But if they are starting to get full, it's time to take one last bite and put the fork down. *It's okay to leave food on the plate!*

I also encourage the families I work with to take their time while eating meals. It takes about 20 minutes for the body to register that it's satisfied. If you finish your meal in less than 20 minutes and are still hungry, wait before eating more. Let the full 20 minutes pass before you reach for the fork again. By then the fullness signal will have reached your brain, and you won't want to continue eating.

Also, help your kids choose foods that increase their sense of fullness—these are generally foods that are high in water and fiber content, such as fruits and vegetables. Eating a piece of fruit can also help satisfy a craving for sweets. Choosing foods that keep you feeling fuller longer is like getting better gas mileage in a car.

There you have it: the rules of the road to help your children lose weight and have fun. Up ahead are delicious road-tested breakfasts, lunches, dinners, snacks, and more. So hop in and let's get going!

3
●●●

HIGH-PERFORMANCE BREAKFASTS

I know you've heard this umpteen times before, but it bears repeating: Breakfast is the most important meal of the day, especially for children. If your kids don't have enough energy to get the day started, they'll feel as if someone has flattened their tires and stuck them in neutral. They'll hit a blood sugar low and crash.

To crashproof your kids, put gas in their bodies first thing in the morning with a healthy breakfast. After 8 hours of sleep, their tummies are on "empty." Eating breakfast refuels your child's body, replenishes blood sugar levels, and revs up the metabolism. And there are even more benefits. Children who eat breakfast:

● Have better concentration, problem-solving skills, and eye-hand coordination. They'll be more alert and creative and less likely to miss days of school. They may even perform better on achievement and standardized tests, have higher grades, and show sharper memories.

● Have lots of energy to play. Breakfast eaters have better muscle strength during the morning.

● Feel less cranky and fatigued.

● Obtain kid-important nutrients like protein and fiber. Fiber, combined with protein, keeps blood sugar from spiking, which can help with appetite and weight control. Breakfast supplies other vital nutrients like calcium and iron.

● Keep their weight under control and are less hungry throughout the day. Breakfast skippers, on the other hand, tend to binge later in the day because they get so hungry. That habit sets them up for obesity—now and in adulthood.

What If Your Kids Hate Breakfast?

Many kids don't like eating breakfast, and it's not an easy job to get them to the breakfast table. One big reason children shun breakfast is that some parents push limited food choices, like oatmeal, every day, and that gets boring. Try offering your kids a variety of breakfast foods: waffles, pancakes, eggs, different cereals, and so forth. Some of the recipes in this chap-ter, like FRUIT PIZZA (page 42) and BREAKFAST BURRITOS (page 45), will help make breakfast more appealing. You don't always have to offer traditional breakfast foods, either. A peanut butter sandwich can make a great breakfast. Any Green Light food your kids enjoy eating in the morning is okay if it gets them to eat breakfast. And if you involve your kids in breakfast decision making, they are more likely to be excited about eating it.

One of my patients, Beth Ann, age 14, never ate breakfast. She gave me every excuse in the book, from not being hungry in the morning to not having enough time to eat. I explained to her that in order to

DETOUR ➡

THE JUICE MYTH

You might think that fruit juice is as healthy as a piece of fruit, but this is what I call the "juice myth." Juice is typically loaded with sugar and is not a good source of fiber. Drinking too much juice may even cause a child to develop a preference for sweet drinks. Children should be encouraged to eat—not drink—the traffic lights in their game plans. Introduce your children to juice in the same way as you'd introduce them to chocolate: at an older age, in small doses, and as a treat—not as a diet staple.

The American Academy of Pediatrics recommends less than 6 ounces of juice a day for children under 6 and less than 12 ounces of juice a day for children ages 7 to 18. I urge my patients to avoid juice completely. I encourage them to eat a piece of fruit instead, which contains the same nutrients, plus fiber. Remember, fresh fruit is **Free Fuel**, while fruit juice counts as a **Green Light**.

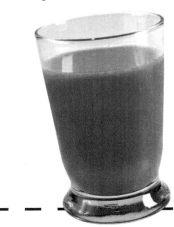

Red Light, Green Light, Eat Right

Check Your Child's Water Level!

Kids must be adequately hydrated to function at their best. Water is crucial for brain function, including concentration and alertness. But how much is enough? Children need to drink 4 to 5 cups of water daily to prevent dehydration. Yet few children drink that much. If their school allows it, send your kids to school with a refillable water bottle that they can sip from whenever they are thirsty. And make sure that your kids have a glass of water with meals and snacks, instead of caffeinated drinks like soda, which dehydrate the body.

lose weight, she had to follow the program. This meant eating breakfast every morning. Although she was resistant, Beth Ann said she would give it a try.

The first week, she grumbled because she felt like she was forcing herself to eat when she wasn't hungry. I assured her that her body would get used to eating in the morning. To save time, I suggested that she plan her breakfast the night before and wake up 10 minutes earlier each morning.

By the end of the second week, Beth Ann was actually looking forward to breakfast! She loved the fact that she was no longer famished by lunchtime. In fact, she reported that she was eating less over the course of the day. "I can't believe that by adding breakfast, I am eating less and feeling less hungry!" she said. She was thrilled, especially when she started losing weight. After 15 weeks, she was down 20 pounds. Children need a good start in the morning, and breakfast is the answer.

Alertness Fuel for School

Food is like gasoline for the body, including the brain. If you feed your kids a nutritionally bankrupt, low-octane breakfast, they'll be running on fumes all morning. If you fuel their tanks with the good stuff, they'll have strong, clean-running engines and will be ready for optimal performance.

Your child's breakfast will consist of the number of Green Lights specified by his or her game plan (see Chapter 2). Adding Free Fuel will help complete a healthy breakfast. Fruit, in particular, makes a great breakfast partner—it contains fiber and is a good source of energy. Here's a look at the top-five breakfast foods that boost brainpower and give kids the energy they need to learn and cope with busy school days.

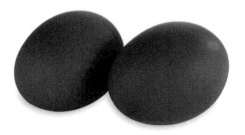

1. Eggs and Egg Whites

🔘 1 egg = 1 **Green Light**

🔘 4 egg whites = 1 **Green Light**

Eggs and egg whites are loaded with protein—a terrific nutrient for brainpower. Protein boosts alertness, which is why you want to make sure your kids have some protein in the morning before they head off to school. Protein also helps kids feel fuller longer, so they won't be starving by their second period class. Children are more active, motivated, and energetic when their breakfast contains healthy protein.

Eggs and egg whites also contain a B vitamin called choline. Choline is another brain booster. Studies show that people perform better on memory tests after eating choline-containing foods.

2. Avocado

🔘 2 ounces avocado = 1 **Green Light**

Avocado for breakfast? You bet! Avocado is packed with boron, a mineral that may increase energy levels and boost brainpower. Studies conducted by the US Department of Agriculture and published in various scientific journals suggest that people with high boron levels perform better on tasks that require attention and memory. Boron also helps stabilize blood sugar levels. A good way to enjoy avocado for breakfast is to add it to omelets. Just remember that avocado is not a **Free Fuel** and must be counted as one of that day's **Green Light** foods.

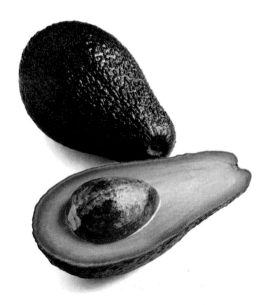

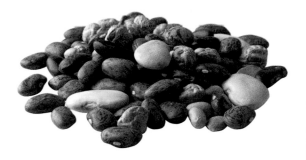

3. Beans

● ¼ cup = 1 **Green Light**

Beans are an excellent source of B vitamins, which help your children think more clearly and feel more energetic. They also offer plenty of fiber. Fiber stabilizes blood sugar, keeps energy level even, and adds bulk to fill your child up. A great way to enjoy beans in the morning is to eat them in a BREAKFAST BURRITO like the one on page 45.

4. Oatmeal

● ¾ cup plain oatmeal, prepared = 1 **Green Light**

Oatmeal is a whole grain, complex carbohydrate

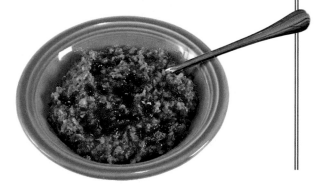

that gives your child energy without causing rapid shifts in insulin (and blood sugar) levels. Complex carbs can decrease anxiety and depression by increasing brain levels of serotonin, the happy chemical. Complex carbs like oatmeal also help make your child more attentive.

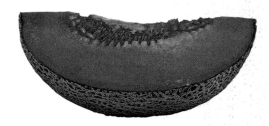

5. Fruit

● Fresh fruit = **Free Fuel**

Breakfast is a good opportunity for your child to eat a serving of fresh fruit. Fruit is a great source of complex carbohydrates, fiber, and antioxidants (which protect brain cells as well as other cells in the body). Some easy ways to incorporate fruit into breakfast include topping cold cereal with a sliced banana, stirring blueberries into hot oatmeal, topping pancakes or waffles with sliced strawberries, or including cantaloupe slices or grapefruit or orange segments on a plate with eggs or toast.

Breakfast Menus to Keep Engines Revved All Day

When planning your child's breakfast, aim for protein, fiber, and calcium. An easy way to meet this objective is to make a Traffic Light Muffin: an egg (**Green Light**) and a slice of fat-free cheese (**Free Fuel**) placed between two halves of a toasted light, whole wheat English muffin (**Green Light**), with some fruit (**Free Fuel**) on the side. Just be sure to cook the egg without added fats or oils or you will need to count each serving of olive oil or butter as a traffic light. I use cooking spray when making my kids' breakfasts. A Traffic Light Muffin is a perfect breakfast because it combines brain-boosting protein, fiber, whole grains, calcium-rich dairy, and fruit. The calcium in the cheese is another "smart nutrient." It promotes clear thinking and focus.

Here are 14 sample breakfast menus, to provide 2 weeks' worth of healthy options. Several of these menus feature recipes you'll find later in this chapter. Also, keep in mind that some children will have fewer or more colors in their plans, so portion sizes will need to be adjusted accordingly. **Choose foods based on the number of colors allotted in your child's personalized meal plan.**

SAMPLE BREAKFASTS

OPTION 1

1 packet low-sugar oatmeal (**Yellow**)

1 apple (**Free Fuel**)

OPTION 2

BANANA DOG (page 36) (**Green, Green**)

OPTION 3

1 cup raisin bran + ½ cup fat-free milk (**Green, Green**)

1 cup mixed berries (**Free Fuel**)

OPTION 4

1 low-fat frozen waffle (**Green**)

Sugar-free syrup (**Free Fuel**)

1 cup fat-free milk (**Green**)

Raspberries (**Free Fuel**)

OPTION 5

1 BREAKFAST QUESADILLA (page 38) (**Yellow**)

Kiwi (**Free Fuel**)

OPTION 6

4 egg whites, scrambled (**Green**) with spinach (**Free Fuel**)

1 slice fat-free cheese (**Free Fuel**)

2 slices Canadian-style bacon (**Green**)

OPTION 7

7 minimuffins of TURKEY PEPPERONI QUICHE (page 39) (**Green**)

Cantaloupe slices (**Free Fuel**)

OPTION 8

3 slices FRENCH TOAST (page 41) (**Green, Green**)

1 pear (**Free Fuel**)

OPTION 9

1 slice FRUIT PIZZA (page 42) (**Yellow**)

Red Light, Green Light, Eat Right

WHEAT BEFORE WHITE

Even though white bread and whole wheat bread are both **Green Light** foods, whole wheat bread is much healthier due to its higher fiber content. White foods—like white bread, white rice, and white pasta, as well as cookies, candies, and cakes made with refined white sugar and flour—are rapidly broken down into sugar (glucose). When kids eat these foods, their blood is quickly flooded with sugar. This causes their blood sugar levels to spike. The body then responds by converting the sugar to fat, causing blood sugar levels to come crashing down. The blood then contains little to no sugar, and your child gets super hungry and is more likely to eat again sooner.

When kids eat whole wheat bread, their blood sugar remain stable. Because whole grains contain fiber and are not as easily broken down into sugar, glucose enters the bloodstream gradually. The sugar is not converted to fat; instead, it remains steady and is burned as energy. It takes a lot longer for hunger to strike again!

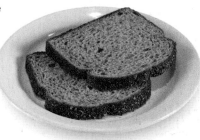

OPTION 10

6 ounces fat-free yogurt, plain (**Green**)

¼ cup low-fat granola (**Green**)

1 cup strawberries (**Free Fuel**)

OPTION 11

2 BREAKFAST BURRITOS (page 45) (**Green, Green**)

½ cup pineapple, canned in its own juice, juice discarded (**Free Fuel**)

OPTION 12

1 fat-free cereal bar (**Green**)

1 tube Go-Gurt (**Green**)

1 cup mixed berries (**Free Fuel**)

OPTION 13

VEGETABLE EGG FRITTATA (page 46) (**Green, Green**)

1 orange (**Free Fuel**)

OPTION 14

4 frozen minipancakes (**Green**)

Sugar-free syrup (**Free Fuel**)

⅔ cup low-fat chocolate milk (**Green**)

2 small clementines (**Free Fuel**)

High-Performance Breakfast Recipes

Here are a number of delicious, easy-to-fix recipes that fit the bill for energy, protein, and overall nutrition. I'm sure they'll inspire some great breakfast ideas of your own. If you are creative and think outside the box, breakfast can be very tasty, and your kids will love it!

Banana Dog

What's more fun than a "hot dog" for breakfast? Kids love this simple, tasty breakfast, and it's easy to eat on the go.

MAKES 1 SERVING ■ EACH SERVING (1 BANANA DOG) = 2 GREENS

PREP TIME: 3 minutes

COOK TIME: None

READY TIME: 3 minutes

1 tablespoon peanut butter

1 light (preferably wheat) hot dog roll

1 banana

2 teaspoons sugar-free jelly

1. Spread the peanut butter on the hot dog roll.

2. Place the banana in the hot dog roll.

3. Spread the sugar-free jelly on the banana.

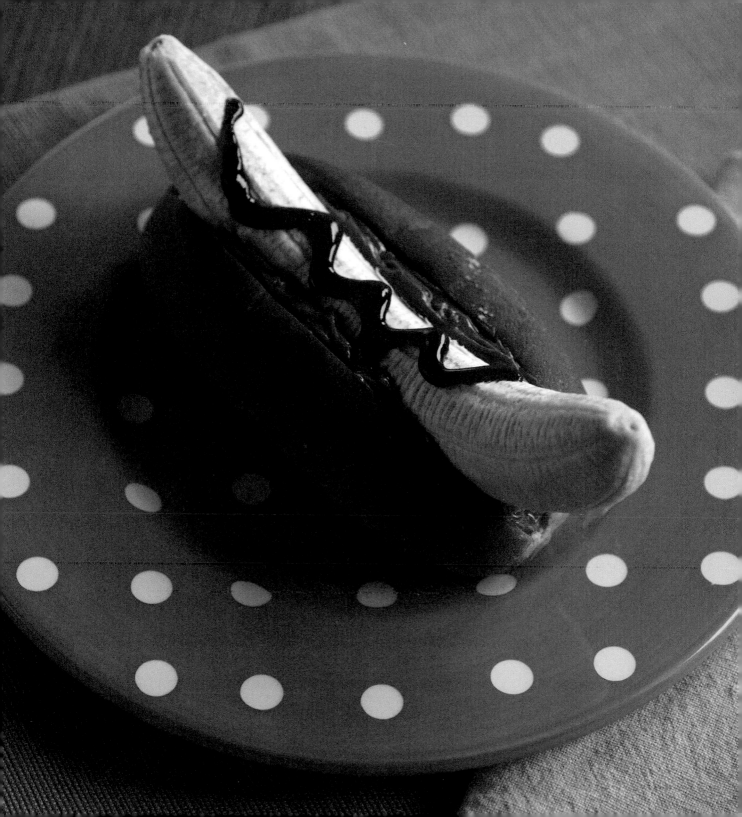

Breakfast Quesadilla

Here's a twist on the usual toast and eggs. It's just as quick to prepare, and your kids can fold it up and eat it with their hands—no utensils required!

MAKES 1 SERVING ■ EACH SERVING = 1 YELLOW

PREP TIME: 5 minutes
COOK TIME: 5 minutes
READY TIME: 10 minutes

Vegetable cooking spray

1 egg

1 (6-inch) wheat tortilla

½ cup shredded fat-free
    Cheddar cheese

2 tablespoons salsa

1. Spray vegetable cooking spray into a frying pan.

2. Scramble the egg and cook to the desired degree of doneness.

3. Cut the tortilla in half.

4. Place the cooked egg on the tortilla half.

5. Sprinkle the cheese over the egg.

6. Place the other tortilla half on top.

7. Microwave for 30 seconds.

8. Spoon the salsa on top.

Turkey Pepperoni Quiche

Turkey pepperoni adds flavor and spice to this quiche with less fat than beef or pork pepperoni. You can freeze these in zip-top bags and then reheat on a cookie sheet.

MAKES 9 DOZEN MINIMUFFINS ■ EACH SERVING (7 MINIMUFFINS) = 1 GREEN

PREP TIME: 15 minutes
COOK TIME: 10–12 minutes
READY TIME: 45 minutes

16 ounces fat-free mozzarella, shredded

1 (6-ounce) container fat-free ricotta

48 "circles" Hormel turkey pepperoni

⅓ cup flour

1 teaspoon baking powder

20 egg whites (or 1¼ cups egg substitute)

⅔ cup fat-free milk

1. Preheat the oven to 325°F.

2. In a large bowl, mix the cheeses, pepperoni, flour, and baking powder.

3. In a separate bowl, whisk together the egg whites and milk.

4. Pour the egg white mixture into the cheese mixture and carefully fold together.

5. Pour the batter into prepared minimuffin pans. Fill each muffin cup about three-quarters full with the quiche mixture.

6. Bake for about 10 to 12 minutes or until set.

7. Carefully loosen and remove the quiches from the muffin tins. Cool on a cooling rack; serve warm.

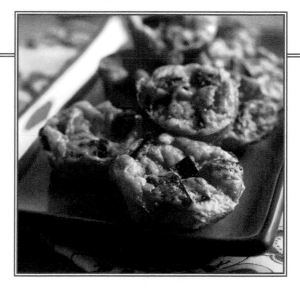

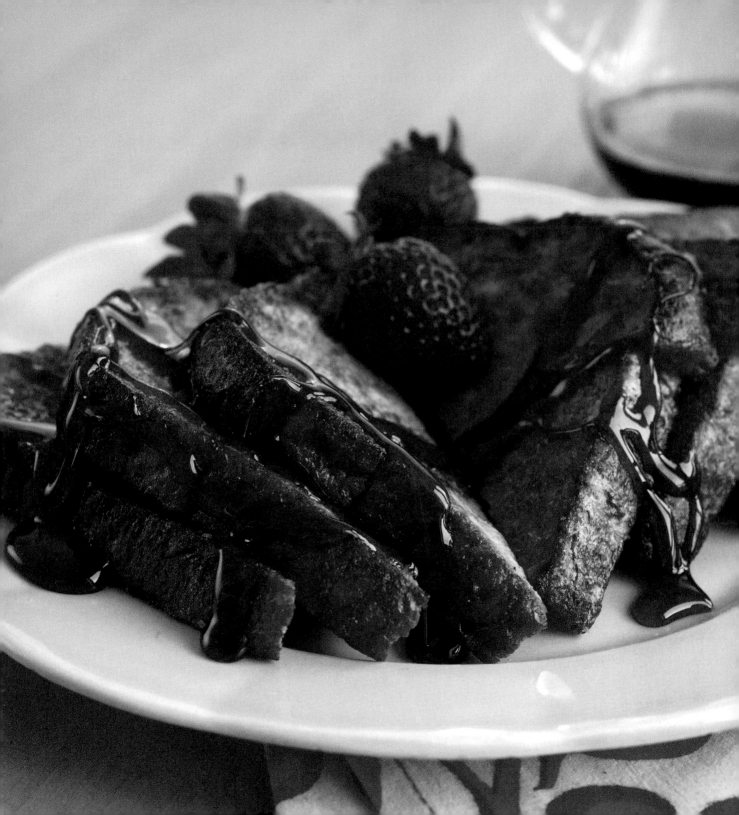

French Toast

There's nothing like the heavenly smell of cinnamon to get your kids out of bed! I make this recipe at home, and it gets rave reviews every time.

MAKES 6 SLICES ■ EACH SERVING (3 SLICES) = 2 GREENS

PREP TIME: **8** minutes
COOK TIME: **4** minutes
READY TIME: **12** minutes

6 egg whites
1 tablespoon vanilla extract
1 cup Splenda
2 tablespoons ground cinnamon
6 slices light whole wheat bread
Vegetable cooking spray
Sugar-free pancake syrup

1. Combine the egg whites and vanilla in a bowl. Gently mix.

2. Combine the Splenda and cinnamon in a second bowl. Gently mix.

3. Place a slice of bread into the egg white mixture and thoroughly coat it on both sides.

4. Place the bread into the Splenda mixture and thoroughly coat it on both sides.

5. Repeat steps 3 and 4 until all slices of bread are fully coated. You may need to make more egg white or Splenda mixture to fully saturate the bread.

6. Spray vegetable cooking spray into a frying pan set over medium-high heat. Allow the oil to heat.

7. Cook the bread in the pan until the egg looks cooked, about 1 to 2 minutes.

8. Flip the bread over and cook another minute or so.

9. Top with sugar-free syrup and enjoy.

Fruit Pizza

If you have a child who is not a breakfast eater, make his morning meal fun by serving a fruit pizza! This is a great recipe for using up any ripe fruit you have in your kitchen—just slice it and toss it on.

MAKES 5 SERVINGS ■ EACH SERVING (1 SLICE, OR ⅕ OF THE PIE) = 1 YELLOW

PREP TIME: 10 minutes

COOK TIME: 10–15 minutes

READY TIME: 25 minutes

12-inch Boboli whole wheat thin-crust pizza dough

2 cups fat-free yogurt

Sliced fruit (apples, grapes, mango, melon, strawberries, blueberries)

1. Preheat the oven to 450°F.

2. Bake the pizza crust on a rack or baking sheet according to package directions.

3. Briefly let the crust cool.

4. Spread the yogurt over the crust.

5. Top with sliced fruit.

6. Cut into 5 slices.

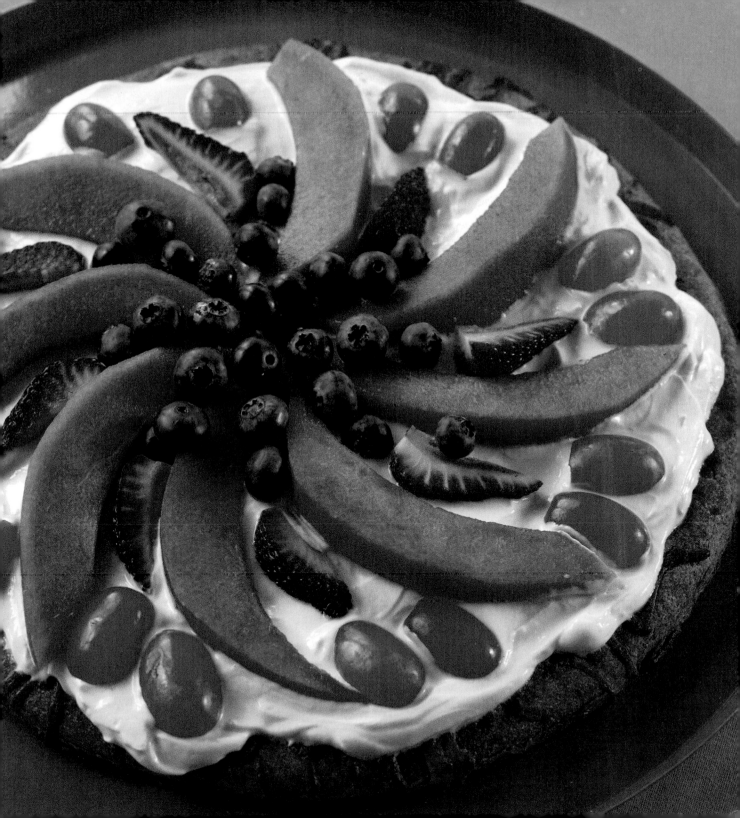

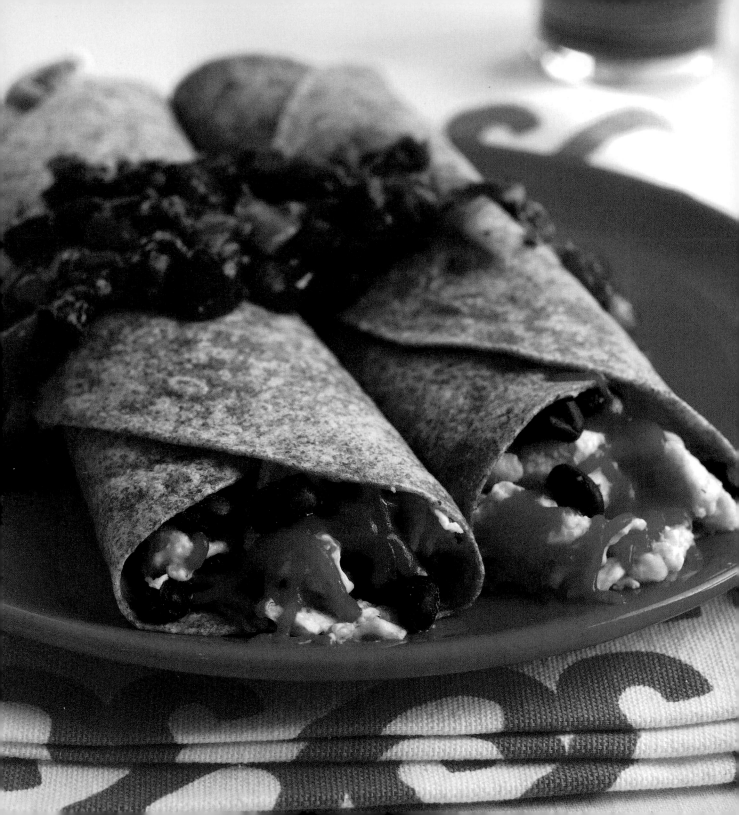

Breakfast Burritos

Using egg whites to replace whole eggs in a recipe is a great way to cut fat and cholesterol. It will also increase the volume of food your kids get to eat.

MAKES 1 SERVING ■ EACH SERVING (2 BURRITOS) = 2 GREENS

PREP TIME: 5 minutes

COOK TIME: 5 minutes

READY TIME: 10 minutes

Vegetable cooking spray

2 egg whites

2 whole wheat tortillas

¼ cup fat-free cheese

¼ cup rinsed canned beans (such as pinto beans or black beans)

Salsa (to taste)

1. Spray vegetable cooking spray into a frying pan.

2. Scramble the egg whites in the pan and cook to the desired degree of doneness.

3. Place the cooked eggs on the tortillas.

4. Sprinkle the cheese over the eggs.

5. Place the beans over the cheese and eggs.

6. Roll each tortilla into a wrap.

7. Microwave for 30 seconds.

8. Spoon salsa on top.

Vegetable Egg Frittata

Here's a breakfast dish that's loaded with Free Fuel!

MAKES 4 SERVINGS ■ EACH SERVING (¼ OF FRITTATA) = 2 GREENS

PREP TIME: 10 minutes
COOK TIME: 20 minutes
READY TIME: 30 minutes

7 eggs

1 tablespoon fresh basil
or 1 teaspoon dried basil,
crushed

Vegetable cooking spray

¾ cup frozen whole kernel corn

½ cup chopped zucchini

⅓ cup thinly sliced scallions
(about 3 scallions)

¾ cup sliced tomatoes (about
2 tomatoes)

½ cup shredded fat-free
Cheddar cheese (2 ounces)

1. Slightly beat the eggs. Add the basil. Set aside.

2. Spray vegetable cooking spray onto a skillet. Add the corn, zucchini, and scallions.

3. Cook the vegetables for 3 minutes, stirring often.

4. Add the tomatoes.

5. Cook, uncovered, over medium heat for about 5 minutes or until the vegetables are tender yet still slightly crunchy, stirring occasionally.

6. Pour the egg mixture over the vegetables. Cook over medium heat.

7. Allow the eggs to cook, being sure to frequently lift eggs slightly to allow the uncooked portion to flow underneath.

8. Continue cooking until the eggs are almost set.

9. Sprinkle the mixture with the cheese.

10. Put the skillet under the oven broiler, 4 to 5 inches from heat.

11. Broil 1 to 2 minutes or until the top is just set and the cheese is melted.

12. Cut into 4 equal pieces while still hot.

High-Performance Breakfasts On the Go

If your family is like mine, your mornings are hectic and often so busy that you barely have enough time to get yourself ready, let alone prepare a nutritious breakfast for everybody else. Don't worry; no one has to miss breakfast because of mad dashes out the door. There are plenty of simple, convenient, and healthy options to start your child's day off on the right foot. Here are my suggestions for quick breakfasts on the go; these can be packed in a backpack and eaten on the bus or before class. Each one is worth two **Greens** (or one **Yellow**) and should be accompanied by **Free Fuel**:

- Fiber One bar
- PowerBar
- Light English muffin, spread with 1 tablespoon peanut butter or almond butter
- Nutri-Grain bar
- 2 soft granola bars
- 2 tubes Go-Gurt yogurt

Here are some other tips to help make your family's morning meal less hectic.

- Plan breakfast the night before. Premeasure portions of cereal in resealable containers or food storage bags and put milk in cups in the fridge.
- I love breakfast bars. Paired with a piece of fruit, they make a quick, nutritious breakfast.
- Maintain a well-stocked pantry and refrigerator. Have plenty of whole grain frozen waffles and pancakes around, as well as packaged cereals and instant oatmeal.
- Make breakfast a priority. If time is limited, wake up 10 to 15 minutes earlier to prepare it.
- Whip up a batch of smoothies and make everyone's breakfast at once. Blend fresh or frozen fruit such as strawberries, pineapple, or bananas with fat-free milk or low-fat yogurt and pour into Thermos-style containers that kids can take on the go.

If your children are on a school breakfast plan or are dropped off early for activities or sports, obtain a copy of the cafeteria menu. If no healthy options are available, pack breakfast for your kids using the suggestions above.

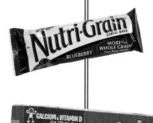

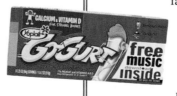

Cut Costs at the Supermarket

It's true that healthy foods often cost a little more than junky foods and fast foods. If you're watching your bottom line, here are some tips to help keep your family budget in good shape.

1. Make three shopping lists.

Write down what you need immediately, what you will need soon, and what you already have. When you get to the supermarket, select the items that you need first. Then look at the list of what you will need soon. Are any of those items on sale? If so, buy them now. If not, wait until next week. Check against the list of items you have on hand to avoid purchasing other foods on sale that you may not need.

2. Don't shop when you or your kids are hungry.

Shopping on an empty stomach will sabotage your waistline and your wallet. Hungry shoppers fill their baskets with all kinds of nonessentials. Have a healthy snack before heading out the door.

3. Buy in bulk.

Consider going to a wholesale store for your nonperishables. Instead of purchasing small packages, look for bigger containers and boxes to save money. To see if you are really getting a better deal, compare the *unit prices* of the bigger and smaller containers on the store's shelf. Then make your own single-serving packages at home. For example, you might buy a large barrel of pretzel rods and portion them into small bags for lunch boxes or car snacks.

4. Buy in season.

Fruit is often reasonably priced when it is bought in season. Take advantage of nature's seasonal bounty. For example:

- SUMMER: blackberries, blueberries, cantaloupe, cherries, honeydew melon, nectarines, peaches, plums, raspberries, strawberries, and watermelon
- FALL: apples, figs, grapes, pears, and pomegranates
- WINTER: bananas, cranberries, grapefruit, lemons, oranges, and tangerines
- SPRING: apricots, mangoes, and pineapple

5. Buy frozen.

If fresh produce is too expensive, consider frozen. Frozen fruits and vegetables contain the same vitamins and nutrients as fresh.

6. Check for sales.

Stock up on nonperishables when they go on sale. Look for the generic or store brand; these are generally cheaper.

7. Use coupons.

Many supermarkets offer coupons. Clip and save them until you need the featured item. In addition to finding coupons the old-fashioned way in your newspaper or store circular, check the Internet—these days, using coupons is practically chic, and several Web sites provide valuable coupons and money-saving strategies.

From Red Light to Green Light!

Once you become familiar with the program, you and your kids will enjoy planning **Green Light** morning meals. One of my patients, Tommy, age 8, told me he and his mom now plan breakfasts and shop for breakfast foods together. He loves going to the grocery store with his mom and pointing out which foods are **Green, Yellow,** and **Red.** In the bread aisle, for instance, Mom picked up a package of bagels, but Tommy knew that one small bagel was a **Yellow.** So Tommy suggested instead that they buy a box of light English muffins. One light English muffin is one **Green Light,** which means that he could pair it with an additional **Green,** such as one egg or four egg whites (one **Green Light**)—a homemade breakfast sandwich. As Tommy and his mother learned, it's easy to take your children's breakfasts from **Red Light** to **Green Light.** Here are some other examples:

BREAKFAST MAKEOVERS

NOT GREAT	BETTER	BEST
2 eggs 2 slices toast 1½ Tbsp butter	2 eggs 2 slices toast No butter	1 egg 2 slices reduced-calorie toast No butter
2 c sugary cereal 1 c whole milk	1½ c nonsugary cereal 1 c whole milk	¾ c nonsugary, high-fiber cereal 1 c fat-free milk
2 frozen waffles ¼ c regular syrup 1½ Tbsp butter	2 frozen waffles ¼ c regular syrup No butter	2 frozen waffles ¼ c sugar-free syrup No butter
2 slices toast 1½ Tbsp butter	2 slices toast 1 Tbsp reduced-calorie margarine	2 slices toast 10 sprays butter spray
Cheese omelet made with 3 eggs and ⅓ c shredded regular Cheddar cheese, and prepared in 1½ Tbsp vegetable oil	Cheese omelet made with 2 eggs and ⅓ c shredded regular Cheddar cheese, and prepared with vegetable cooking spray	Cheese omelet made with 2 eggs and ½ c shredded fat-free Cheddar cheese, and prepared with vegetable cooking spray

Now that you and your children are on the road to better eating, here's a fun quiz you can take together. It's "open book," too! Feel free to check the database in the back of this book if you're unsure of your answers.

1. If you're planning breakfast and want a muffin, which of the following would be the better (**Green Light**) choice?
   A. 2 minimuffins
   B. 100-calorie pack of muffins
   C. 1 large muffin

2. Cocoa, homemade or store bought, is a **Green Light** food.
   A. True
   B. False

3. You and your kids decide to have breakfast at a fast-food restaurant. Of the three menu items listed below, which one would be the best choice?
   A. Burger King Biscuit—bacon, egg, and cheese (1 sandwich)
   B. Burger King Croissan'wich—bacon, egg, and cheese (1 sandwich)
   C. McDonald's Sausage McMuffin (1 sandwich)

4. You're going grocery shopping and want to pick up some bagels. Of the choices below, which would be the best (**Green Light**) choice?
   A. Small plain bagel
   B. Large whole wheat bagel
   C. Mini cinnamon raisin bagel

5. How many slices of bacon count as a **Green Light**?
   A. 3 slices
   B. 2 slices
   C. No slices; bacon is not a **Green Light** food.

Breakfast is the first step toward feeling good, losing weight, and staying healthy. It gives kids the energy they need to excel in school. Now that you have some creative breakfast ideas and you know how to make them quickly, make eating breakfast a priority in your household!

(Answers: 1—B; 2—B; 3—B; 4—C; 5—B)

4

• • •

MID-MORNING POWER SNACKS

When 11-year-old Liza first came to see me, she proudly told me that she "never snacks," and she eats only breakfast, lunch, and dinner. This didn't surprise me, since snacking has taken on such negative connotations in our society, probably because of all the fattening junk foods available as snacks. So it's no wonder that many people think snacking will pack on pounds. But nothing could be further from the truth.

Snacking doesn't cause weight gain, but allowing your body to get too hungry does. If kids avoid snacks, they may be confronted with ravenous hunger (hungry as a wolf) later on. That's when they'll inevitably overeat the wrong foods. Planned, healthy snacks prevent extreme hunger and reduce the risk of out-of-control eating.

Snacking is thus an important part of weight loss and healthy weight maintenance. Liza was shocked when I told her that she needed to start eating two healthy snacks a day. "How can eating more help me lose weight?" she asked.

I told her that when she becomes too hungry, her blood sugar gets low, which leaves her feeling famished and tired. I explained that snacking increases energy levels, boosts metabolism, and curbs hunger pangs—so she'd end up eating less at each meal. By adding snacks to her day, she wouldn't be eating more; she'd just be eating differently—in a way that would make her body a calorie-burning engine. At first, Liza wasn't convinced, but she said she'd give it a try anyway.

According to her mom, Liza's eyes lit up when she had her first morning snack of whole grain crackers and fat-free cheese. She especially loved her afternoon snack of 94 percent fat-free microwave popcorn. "I feel like I'm cheating," she said. "And it's so great to be able to eat with my friends after school. I used to sit and watch them snack. It was torture. Now I feel like one of the group!"

But the best part of snacking was that Liza lost 2 pounds the first week she implemented regular snacks. "I never thought I would lose weight by adding snacks, but it happened!" And it kept happening. Liza has been on the plan for 7 months. In the first 5 months, she lost 20 pounds and achieved her goal weight, and she has been on the maintenance plan ever since. Liza learned a valuable lesson that I hope will stay with her for life: Healthy snacking helps accelerate weight loss.

While many schools give kids a "snack time," unfortunately, some other schools don't permit snacking. If your kids aren't allowed snacks at school, or if they're older or can't eat in between classes, simply add their morning snack to a different snack or meal. If they have an early lunch, add an extra snack between lunch and dinner. Snacking can be easily adapted to any situation.

$mart Snacking

Your child's morning snack should be a wholesome combination of protein and fiber to stabilize blood sugar and help keep your child feeling full until lunchtime. Most kids like eating a junky snack after school but are more receptive to a healthier morning snack, so this is a good time for incorporating **Green Lights** and **Free Fuel** into their diet. Snacks are always a great opportunity to add nutrients like calcium from fat-free cheese and fat-free or low-fat yogurt.

Most kids get hungry every 3 to 4 hours. Help your children use the Kids' Hunger Scale in Chapter 2 to gauge when their appetite level is between a 2 (hungry as a horse) and a 3 (hungry as a bear). This is the right time for snacking.

Adding snacks to your child's day doesn't mean you have to add to the family food budget. Here are some affordable foods that make delicious, filling morning snacks.

- Vitamin-rich vegetables can become the centerpiece of a morning snack without putting a dent in your wallet. Try broccoli, carrots, cauliflower, cucumbers, celery, and bell peppers with salsa or a fat-free yogurt as a dip. These veggies range from 79 cents to $3 for a supply that will last for many snacks.

The Cheese Stands Alone as a Tooth Protector!

Did you know that cheese protects and strengthens teeth? Like the rest of the body, the mouth depends on overall good nutrition to stay healthy. In fact, our mouths are highly sensitive to poor nutrition, which can

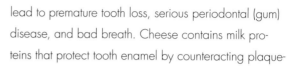

lead to premature tooth loss, serious periodontal (gum) disease, and bad breath. Cheese contains milk proteins that protect tooth enamel by counteracting plaque-causing acids. These acids dissolve minerals inside the enamel crystals of teeth in a process called demineralization. Teeth also regain minerals in a process called remineralization. By delivering minerals to the tooth surface, cheese and other dairy foods promote remineralization.

- Morning snack time is also a convenient time for fruit that travels easily in backpacks, like apples, pears, bananas, and grapes. Fruit makes for an inexpensive snack: A banana can cost as little as 30 cents, and a 3-pound bag of apples often sells for less than $5.

- Low-fat and fat-free dairy foods are excellent sources of protein and calcium. Some dairy foods can also be high in fat and calories, so focus on the choices that are healthiest for your kids: fat-free milk, low-fat or fat-free yogurt, low-fat or fat-free cottage cheese, and low-fat or fat-free cheese. Like milk, cheese contains many essential nutrients, such as protein, calcium, phosphorus, zinc, vitamin A, riboflavin, and vitamin B_{12}.

- Leftovers make terrific snacks. When you make multiple servings of a meal, you'll save money and time. The trick is to plan in advance so that nothing goes to waste. Get creative; a half serving left over from yesterday's OVEN-FRIED CHICKEN lunch (page 78) can be wrapped in half of a whole grain tortilla for a great high-protein snack!

- Low-sodium soup is a low-cost, low-calorie superhero. Sipping on soup will fill up your child without emptying your pockets. A large 14.5-ounce can may sell for as little as 80 cents.

- Nuts and seeds are nutrient-packed snacks. Because nuts are high in fat and calories, many people believe they are unhealthy. However, the fat in nuts is "good fat" that decreases the risk of

⬧ CAUTION ⬧ NUT ALLERGIES

I strongly caution parents and teachers not to give nuts to children under the age of 2—for two reasons.

First, young children's immune systems have not yet matured, and nuts could trigger an allergic reaction. Nut allergies occur when the body perceives nut protein as a harmful foreign body and reacts excessively to combat the invader. The most common nut allergy is to peanuts, but sufferers may also be allergic to other nuts. If you have a strong family history of nut or peanut allergy, wait until your children are 3 years old before introducing nuts into their diets. If a child does have an allergy, contact your child's teacher and school food workers to let them know that your child's food cannot come in contact with nuts or be prepared with equipment that has touched nuts. If your child's allergy is especially severe, you're probably safest packing his or her lunch. It's also important to instruct your child not to share food with friends or eat any food at class parties that you haven't preapproved.

Second, nuts can be a choking hazard, so make sure your kids are old enough to chew and eat them without the likelihood of choking. Regardless of age, children should be sitting down and under adult supervision while eating nuts.

heart disease. These essential fats, called omega-3 and omega-6 fats, are vital for growth, healthy skin and hair, blood pressure control, immunity, and healthy cholesterol levels. Essential fatty acids also play a key role in healthy brain development. Nuts are one of the best natural sources of vitamin E, magnesium, potassium, folate, copper, and selenium. In the right portion, they are a great food for weight control. Nuts are filling due to their protein, fat, and fiber content. In studies, volunteers lost weight when they ate nuts in conjunction with a healthy, balanced diet.

A serving size of nuts is 1 ounce, which is equivalent to a palmful. Also, ⅓ cup of nuts is equal to 1 ounce of meat. Because nuts are calorie dense, moderation and portion control are key, especially if your child is trying to lose weight. The chart on the opposite page lists healthy serving sizes for nuts. Each variety of nut counts as a **Green Light,** except for Brazil nuts, which are a **Yellow Light.**

SERVING SIZE AND TRAFFIC LIGHT VALUES FOR NUTS AND SEEDS

ALMONDS	12 almonds	🔴
BRAZIL NUTS	6 Brazil nuts	🔴
CASHEWS	7 cashews	🔴
HAZELNUTS	10 hazelnuts	🔴
MACADAMIA NUTS	5 macadamia nuts	🔴
MIXED NUTS, DRY ROASTED	2 Tbsp	🔴
PEANUTS	20 peanuts	🔴
PEANUT BUTTER, REGULAR OR REDUCED FAT	1 Tbsp	🔴
PECANS	6 pecan halves	🔴
PISTACHIOS	20 pistachios or 2 Tbsp	🔴
PUMPKIN SEEDS, WITHOUT SHELLS	2 Tbsp	🔴
SUNFLOWER SEEDS, WITH SHELLS	1/3 c	🔴
SUNFLOWER SEEDS, WITHOUT SHELLS	2 Tbsp	🔴
TRAIL MIX, +/− CHOCOLATE	2 Tbsp	🔴
WALNUTS	6 walnut halves	🔴

Mending Vending

Many kids buy snack foods at vending machines located on school property. Most items in these machines are not very healthy, though some districts and states have started to regulate what kinds of vending machines are allowed on public school grounds. I generally encourage children not to rely on vending machines for their daily snacks unless they are old enough and comfortable enough to consistently make healthy choices.

The good news is, there *are* some healthy options in vending machines. Tucked between empty-calorie items, there may be fat-free milk, water, yogurt, trail mix, whole grain crackers, granola bars, or nuts. But the portions are generally quite large, so if your child selects a snack from the vending machine, he or she will probably need to count out the correct serving size of nuts, crackers, pretzels, and so forth. When it comes to beverages, kids should avoid sodas, iced teas, juices, punches, and sports drinks. These items are loaded with sugar and calories and will interfere with weight loss. Your best bet is to have your kids carry their own snacks so they can avoid the temptation of the vending machine.

NAVIGATING LABEL LANGUAGE

Do you ever feel confused by all of the different health claims you read on the front of packaged foods? What do they actually mean? It's important to understand label language because it can be very misleading. For instance, if a product is labeled as "reduced fat" or "light," it may still contain a significant amount of fat. Take potato chips as an example. To be called "reduced fat," chips must have 25 percent less fat than regular potato chips. To be called "light," chips must have 50 percent less fat than regular potato chips. But there are no set limits on how much fat a "reduced fat" or "light" chip must contain. Always rely on the nutrition facts label rather than on advertising claims like "reduced fat" or "light." Here are some common claims and their meanings, according to FDA regulations.

● **REDUCED FAT.** This term means that a food product contains at least 25 percent less fat than the regular, or comparison, product.

● **LIGHT OR "LITE."** The food contains 50 percent less fat than is contained in the comparison food. The term "light" is also sometimes used to describe food properties such as texture and color. Make sure you understand what information is being conveyed and read the nutrition facts label.

● **LESS FAT.** This term means a food, whether altered or not, contains 25 percent less fat than the comparison food. For example, pretzels that have 25 percent less fat than potato chips could carry a "less" claim.

● **FAT FREE.** The food contains less than 0.5 gram of fat *per serving*.

● **LOW FAT.** This term means a product has less than 3 grams of fat *per serving*.

● **LEAN AND EXTRA-LEAN.** These terms can be used to describe the fat content of meat, poultry, and fish. "Lean" means the product is 90 percent fat free and contains 10 grams or less of fat, 4.5 grams or less of saturated fat, and less than 95 milligrams of cholesterol per serving and per 100 grams. "Extra-lean" proteins are 93 percent fat free, which means they contain 5 grams or less of fat, less than 2 grams of saturated fat, and less than 95 milligrams of cholesterol per serving and per 100 grams. I recommend buying extra-lean meats whenever possible.

What's for a (Morning) Snack?

Mid-morning snacks don't have to be complicated. A simple piece of fruit combined with a container of yogurt is easy to pack in a backpack and will give your child the energy he needs. Here are 14 simple, portable morning snack ideas, along with their traffic light values.

SAMPLE MORNING SNACKS

OPTION 1

1 reduced-calorie granola bar (**Green**)

1 medium peach (**Free Fuel**)

OPTION 2

1 container of Danimals yogurt (**Green**)

1 apple (**Free Fuel**)

OPTION 3

12 almonds (**Green**)

1 medium pear (**Free Fuel**)

OPTION 4

Small box of raisins (**Green**)

1 orange (**Free Fuel**)

OPTION 5

1 serving GORP (page 59) (**Yellow**)

1 medium apple (**Free Fuel**)

OPTION 6

100-calorie pack muffins (**Green**)

1 medium Chinese pear (**Free Fuel**)

OPTION 7

2 rice cakes, flavored (**Green**)

1 serving BOILED EDAMAME (page 59) (**Free Fuel**)

OPTION 8

40 Goldfish crackers (**Green**)

1 cup TROPICAL FRUIT SALAD (page 60) (**Free Fuel**)

OPTION 9

12 light tortilla chips (**Green**)

Salsa (**Free Fuel**)

OPTION 10

1 reduced-fat string cheese (**Green**)

1 cup grapes (**Free Fuel**)

OPTION 11

10 Wheat Thins (**Green**)

1 slice fat-free cheese (**Free Fuel**)

1 medium apple (**Free Fuel**)

OPTION 12

1 serving CREAM OF VEGETABLE SOUP (page 63) (**Green**)

1 medium orange (**Free Fuel**)

OPTION 13

Honey braided pretzel twists (7 twists) (**Green**)

1 banana (**Free Fuel**)

OPTION 14

1 GREEN LIGHT CHOCOLATE CHIP BROWNIE (page 64) (**Green**)

1 large plum (**Free Fuel**)

TRAFFIC TIP

Calcium

It's important for children and teens to consume low-fat and fat-free dairy products, which contain bone-building calcium and other vital nutrients. I recommend three servings of dairy each day. According to the American Academy of Pediatrics, most kids aren't meeting their daily calcium requirements. Here is the breakdown by age:

Ages 1 to 3: 500 mg a day

Ages 4 to 8: 800 mg a day

Ages 9 to 18: 1,300 mg a day

But what if your child is lactose intolerant or has a dairy allergy?

Children and teens who are lactose intolerant may choose products such as lactose-free milk or take lactase enzyme supplements prior to consuming dairy.

Cheese, especially aged cheese such as Cheddar or Swiss, has almost no lactose. Lactose-intolerant people can usually tolerate moderate amounts of these cheeses without difficulty. The American Academy of Pediatrics recommends that lactose-intolerant children include these cheeses in their diet.

Kids who are allergic to milk and dairy products can obtain calcium from numerous nondairy foods, including fortified cereals, soy products, figs, sardines, tofu, collards, salmon (canned), spinach, fortified oatmeal, kale, rhubarb, canned clams, and rainbow trout.

If your children are not receiving enough calcium from their diet, consider giving them a calcium supplement. Most children's multivitamins don't supply enough of this vital mineral.

Below is a list of calcium-containing foods. Encourage your kids to get their daily calcium from these sources.

DAIRY PRODUCTS

Fat-free yogurt: 1 cup, 490 mg

Fat-free milk: 1 cup, 300 mg

Reduced-fat milk: 1 cup, 300 mg

Swiss cheese: 1 ounce, 270 mg

Mozzarella, part skim: 1 ounce, 210 mg

Frozen yogurt: 1 cup, 200 mg

Ice cream, light: ½ cup, 200 mg

Cottage cheese: 1 cup, 160 mg

Pudding, prepared: ½ cup, 150 mg

Parmesan cheese, grated: 2 tablespoons, 140 mg

American cheese: 1 ounce, 140 mg

NONDAIRY AND FORTIFIED FOODS

Waffle, fortified: 1,150 mg

Soy milk, fortified: 1 cup, 400 mg

Fortified cereal: 1 cup, 300 mg

Canned salmon with bones: 3 ounces, 180 mg

Soybeans, cooked: 1 cup, 180 mg

Almonds: 2 ounces, 150 mg

Navy beans: 1 cup, 130 mg

Spinach, cooked: ½ cup, 130 mg

Black beans: 1 cup, 120 mg

Kale, cooked: ½ cup, 90 mg

Tofu: 1 cup, 40 mg

Broccoli, cooked: ½ cup, 20 mg

Morning Snack Recipes

When you make your kids' snacks at home, you know exactly what they're eating. I've created some basic recipes for morning snacks that are a cinch to pull together and that your kids will love.

Gorp

This is a healthier version of trail mix—a cinch to assemble and fun to eat.

MAKES 3 SERVINGS ■ EACH SERVING = 1 YELLOW

PREP TIME: 8 minutes
COOK TIME: None
READY TIME: 8 minutes

1 ounce (1 palmful) chopped nuts

1½ cups Puffins cereal

½ cup chopped dried fruit

1. Mix all ingredients together.

2. Divide evenly and place in 3 plastic sandwich bags.

Boiled Edamame (Soybeans)

Kids love to eat with their fingers. Edamame is a wonderful peel-and-eat treat!

MAKES MANY SERVINGS ■ EACH SERVING = *FREE FUEL*

PREP TIME: 2 minutes
COOK TIME: 5 minutes
READY TIME: 7 minutes

3 quarts water

1 teaspoon salt, plus more to taste

2 pounds frozen soybeans
    (edamame) in pods

1. In a 5- to 6-quart pan over high heat, bring the water and salt to a boil.

2. Add the frozen soybeans in pods and cook for about 5 minutes, or until beans inside pods are tender to bite (break a pod open to test).

3. Drain and sprinkle with additional salt to taste.

4. Serve warm or cover and chill up to 4 hours.

Tropical Fruit Salad

This Free Fuel salad looks as good as it tastes.

MAKES APPROXIMATELY 6 SERVINGS ■ EACH SERVING (1 CUP) = *FREE FUEL*

PREP TIME: 20 minutes
COOK TIME: None
READY TIME: 20 minutes

2 cups (1-inch) cubed fresh
    pineapple

1 cup peeled and chopped
    papaya or mango

1 cup sliced and peeled
    kiwifruit (approximately
    3 kiwifruit)

1 cup red seedless grapes

⅔ cup (¼-inch-thick) slices
    carambola (star fruit;
    approximately 1)

Sprinkle of sweetened coconut

1 tablespoon honey

2 tablespoons fresh lime juice

1. Combine the pineapple, papaya or mango, kiwifruit, grapes, carambola, and coconut in a medium bowl; chill in the refrigerator for at least 30 minutes.

2. Combine the honey and lime juice in a small bowl; toss with the chilled fruit just before serving.

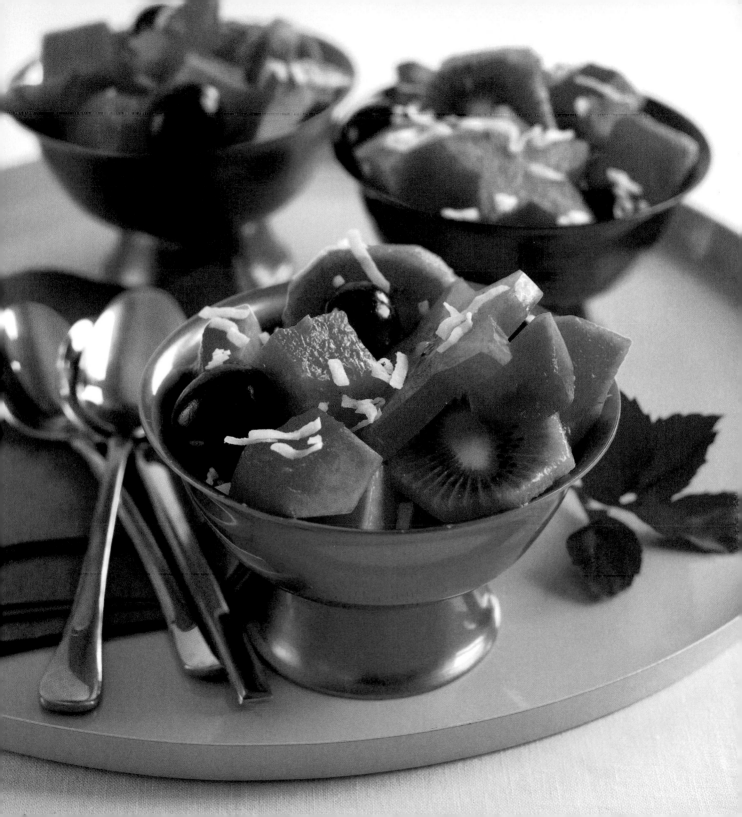

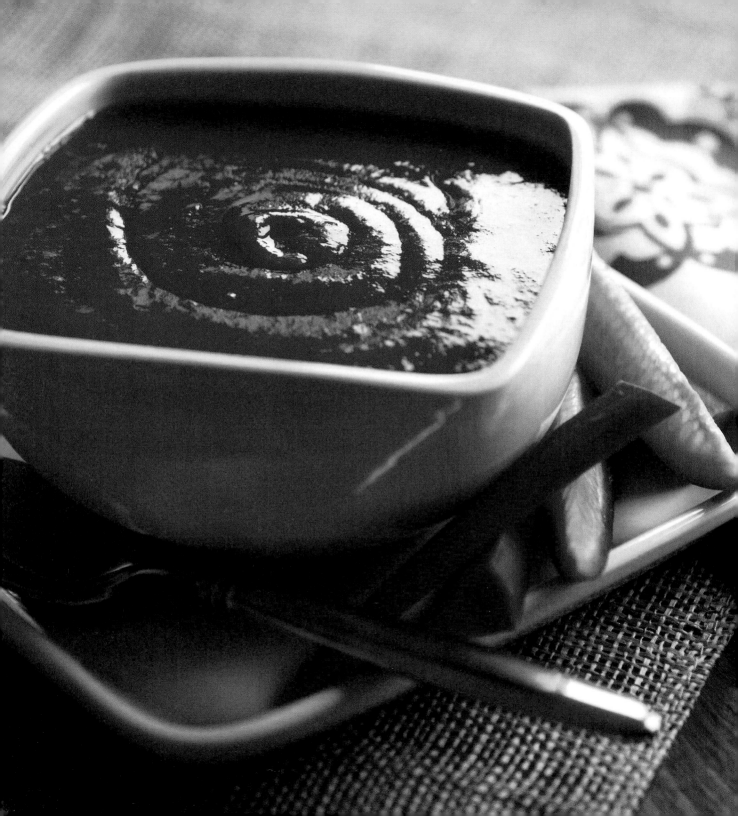

Cream of Vegetable Soup

Soup is one of the best ways to fill up and control appetite. Here's a recipe that supplies plenty of veggies and healthy carbs.

MAKES 4 SERVINGS ■ EACH SERVING (2 CUPS) = 1 GREEN

PREP TIME: 20 minutes
COOK TIME: 40 minutes
READY TIME: 60 minutes

28 ounces fat-free, salt-free chicken broth

3 garlic cloves, minced

2½ cups coarsely chopped onion (about 1 large onion)

1 large baking potato, peeled and cut into 8 (1-inch) pieces

3 large carrots, peeled and cut into 6 pieces

5 medium zucchini, cut into 10 pieces

1 teaspoon salt

¼ teaspoon ground black pepper

⅓ cup half-and-half

1 tablespoon chopped fresh dill

1. Combine the first 6 ingredients in a Dutch oven placed over medium-high heat. Bring to a boil; cover, reduce the heat, and simmer 20 minutes.

2. Place a third of the vegetable mixture in a blender; process until smooth. Repeat the procedure with the remaining vegetable mixture.

3. Return the pureed mixture to the pan. Add the salt, pepper, half-and-half, and dill.

4. Cook over medium heat until thoroughly heated, stirring occasionally. Serve immediately.

Green Light Chocolate Chip Brownies

The families I work with are surprised when they find out they can still eat foods like brownies—and they love this recipe. The coffee granules really bring out the flavor of the chocolate.

MAKES 24 BROWNIES ■ EACH SERVING (1 BROWNIE) = 1 GREEN

PREP TIME: 20 minutes
COOK TIME: 50 minutes
READY TIME: 1 hour 10 minutes

Vegetable cooking spray

16 whole chocolate graham crackers

2 tablespoons unsweetened cocoa powder

¼ teaspoon salt

2 eggs

1 egg white

⅓ cup packed light brown sugar

3 tablespoons Splenda

2 teaspoons instant coffee granules

3 teaspoons vanilla extract

⅔ cup chopped pitted dates

5 tablespoons semisweet chocolate chips

1. Preheat the oven to 300°F. Coat an 8 x 11½-inch baking dish with cooking spray.

2. Using a food processor, crush the graham crackers into crumbs. You should have about 2 cups of crumbs.

3. Transfer the cracker crumbs to a small bowl; add the cocoa and salt and mix well.

4. Combine the eggs, egg white, sugar, and Splenda in a large bowl.

5. Beat the egg mixture with an electric mixer at high speed until thickened, about 2 minutes.

6. Blend in the coffee granules and vanilla.

7. Gently fold in the dates, chocolate chips, and crumb mixture.

8. Scrape the batter into the prepared baking dish, spreading evenly.

9. Bake the brownies until the top springs back when lightly touched, 25 to 30 minutes.

10. Let the brownies cool completely in the pan on a wire rack before cutting.

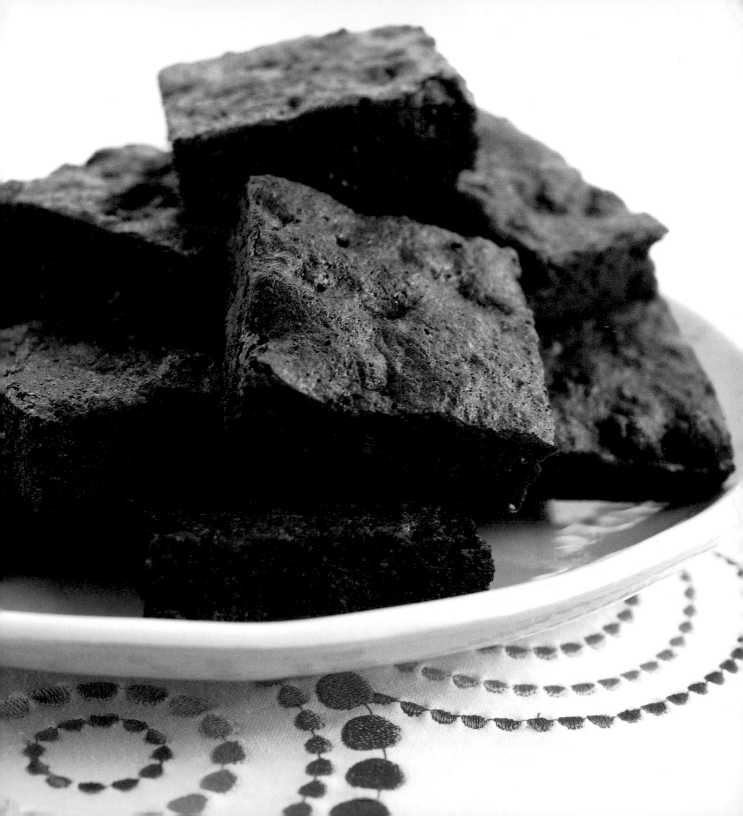

Once you've established a healthy snack plan, your children will eat snacks and enjoy their higher energy level. So get your kids off to the right start in life by adopting healthy snack habits. And don't forget to practice what you preach!

SNACKING AND SODIUM

Many kids' snacks like chips and cookies are packed with salt, a dietary mineral made mostly of sodium chloride. Eating too much salt can raise the body's blood pressure in some people. Often called the "silent killer" because it has no symptoms, high blood pressure (hypertension) increases the risk for stroke, heart attack, heart failure, and kidney failure. High salt intake may even be a risk factor for osteoporosis, according to a 2009 study published in the *Journal of Human Hypertension*.[1] Too much sodium reduces the amount of calcium the body retains, decreasing bone density and increasing the risk for fractures. Although high blood pressure is usually considered an adult disease, pediatricians like me are seeing it more often in kids and teens.

According to the American Heart Association, healthy American adults should eat less than 2,300 milligrams of sodium a day. This is the amount of sodium in just 1 teaspoon of salt! Children need even less sodium in their diets. Here is a list of recommended sodium limits based on your child's age.

Ages 2 to 3: 1,000 mg a day   Ages 9 to 18: 1,500 mg a day

Ages 4 to 8: 1,200 mg a day   Age 19+: 2,300 mg a day

Try to buy low-sodium foods whenever you can. Generally, foods with less than 140 milligrams of sodium per serving are considered low in sodium. These foods will help your kids feel better because they reduce excess fluid in their bodies. But be sure to read labels when you buy packaged foods that advertise reduced- or low-sodium content: Sometimes extra sugar is added to replace the missing salt.

Here are some other useful tips to help you lower your family's sodium intake.

- Fast foods generally contain large amounts of sodium. Try to avoid these foods as much as possible.
- Learn to use herbs, spices, and salt-free seasonings to add flavor to food.
- Fresh is always better when buying meats and vegetables. Frozen is the next best option. Canned goods usually contain large amounts of sodium.
- Use low-sodium baking powder for baking.

5

● ● ●

LUNCHES THAT MAKE THE GRADE

From the first day a child goes to kindergarten to the last day of high school, we as parents trust the school system to nourish our children in mind and body. Yet school lunches generally get poor marks in nutrition and actually contribute to our nation's childhood obesity epidemic. The typical school lunch is short on fresh fruits and veggies and heavy on processed, breaded, and fried entrées. Children are fed foods such as chicken nuggets, french fries, and pepperoni pizza—all high-fat foods that tend to weigh heavily in the digestive tract and may cause drowsiness. Also, kids often consume too much salt and sugar from school lunches, and these ingredients can lead to high blood pressure and obesity.

In addition to keeping up with my medical practice, I'm active within my community to help promote healthier meals at school. I have approached numerous local school boards and politicians in my area about instituting healthier lunch programs. If your child's school lunch isn't making the grade, talk to your food-service director and share your concerns. We parents need to make our voices heard if we are going to resolve the issue of poor nutrition being served to our children.

I suggest to parents that they do not allow their kids to purchase school lunches without first checking the menu. On some days, healthy items may be available, and if your child prefers buying his or her lunch, that's fine. But on days when the unhealthiest items are served, encourage your children to BYOL—"bring your own lunch"—and make it nutritious.

BYOLs can have a great impact on your children's nutrition. Kids who eat wholesome lunches appear to learn better in the afternoon and have higher energy and self-esteem. Even kids who prefer cafeteria lunches of nachos or pizza adapt easily to healthier options when healthy foods are made a consistent part of their routine. Let your child help choose the foods for his or her lunch. Kids are more likely to eat foods that they have helped choose and prepare.

Not Cool to Bring Lunch to School?

Sometimes, kids are embarrassed to bring a healthy lunch to school, or they don't want to call attention to being on a diet. I remember a patient named Aaron, who was about 15 pounds overweight for his size and age. He dug in his heels and refused to BYOL because he was afraid he'd get teased. Here's what I suggested to Aaron: Anytime a classmate asked him why he was bringing his lunch, he should just say, "School lunches are disgusting." Aaron liked the idea, so that's how he responded to questions about his lunch. "I don't like school lunch. It's gross," he said. "The lunch my mom makes tastes better."

This type of response takes the focus off the child and puts it on the school lunch. To Aaron's surprise, the other kids just said, "Oh, okay," and moved on to another subject. And sure enough, over the next few days, his friends started asking him for parts of his lunch. "Can I have your yogurt?" "Hey, I want to share your 100-calorie pack of Doritos!" By the end of the month, his friends were bringing lunch, too. The end result was amazing: Not only did Aaron lose weight, but his entire group of friends was eating healthier!

If your kids don't want to brown-bag every day, I suggest you sit down with them to review the school lunch menu. Allow them to pick one day to buy their favorite meal. Just be sure to remind them: If they eat a **Red Light** food, they must count it as one of their two pit stops for the week!

School Lunch Strategies

Not long ago, I began working with 11-year-old Terri, who was a friendly, outgoing girl. She wasn't obese, but she was overweight by about 16 pounds. Unfortunately, one of her bad habits was eating large portions of her school's cafeteria food. She just couldn't understand why school lunches were so unhealthy.

We obtained a copy of the menu and went through it together. We wrote down the color value of each component of each meal. When she could see the colors in front of her, Terri finally understood what I had been trying to tell her. Here is an example of one of the options on Terri's school menu—a sloppy joe.

SLOPPY JOE

- Roll: **Yellow**
- Ground meat: about ¾ cup: **Yellow** + **Green**
- Sauce: **Free Fuel**
- Corn: about ¾ cup: **Green**

Terri's weight-loss plan allowed for three **Greens** at lunch. This meal "cost" two **Yellows** and two **Greens**. It was way too much!

Like Terri, some kids need to have the menus broken down by color so that they really understand the impact of cafeteria food on their eating plan. Use the Appendix at the back of the book to help you analyze and evaluate the traffic light values on your child's cafeteria menu. School menus vary greatly from district to district, but here's a look at how some typical lunches stack up, based on their color values.

MONDAY
ENTRÉE (choice of one)

- Spicy chicken on wheat bun: 3 ounces spicy chicken (**Yellow**) on wheat bun (**Yellow**)
- Fish fillet on wheat bun: 3 ounces fish fillet (**Yellow**) on wheat bun (**Yellow**)
- PB&J sandwich: 2 slices bread (**Yellow**), 2 tablespoons jelly (**Green**), and 2 tablespoons peanut butter (2 **Greens**)

SIDES (choice of one)

- Seasoned potato wedges: ¾ cup (**Yellow**)
- Green beans, celery and baby carrots, pears, steamed broccoli, chilled peaches, zucchini sticks, cucumber (**Free Fuel**)
- Dip: 1 tablespoon (**Green**)
- Frozen fruit bar: 1 bar (**Yellow**)
- Fruit sherbet: ½ cup (**Yellow**)

TUESDAY
ENTRÉE (choice of one)

- Mac and cheese with muffin: ½ cup pasta (**Yellow**) and ½ large muffin (**Yellow**)
- Turkey corn dog with muffin (**Yellow** + **Green**)

SIDES (choice of one)

- Vegetarian baked beans: ½ cup (**Green**)
- Applesauce: ½ cup (**Green**)
- Orange (**Free Fuel**)
- Raisins: ¼ cup or small box (**Green**)

WEDNESDAY
ENTRÉE (choice of one)

- Soft beef taco with shredded cheese: 1½ tortillas (**Green**) and ⅔ cup beef (**Yellow**)
- Chicken fillet on wheat bun: whole sandwich (**Red**)

SIDES (choice of one)

- Corn on the cob: 1 piece (**Green**)
- Pickles: 2 (**Free Fuel**)
- Lettuce, fruit salad (**Free Fuel**)
- Fruit crisp (**Yellow**)

PIZZA LINE

The "pizza line" is available almost daily in many schools—and it's a very popular option, especially among older kids. Here are the traffic light values for several typical cafeteria pizza options.

- Stuffed crust pizza—cheese and pepperoni: 1 slice (Red)
- Pan pizza—cheese and pepperoni: 1 slice (Yellow + Green)
- Uno pizza wedge—cheese and pepperoni: 1 slice (Red)
- Garlic French bread pizza: 1 slice (Red)

As a once-a-week treat, the pizza line may be okay, but it should not be a daily choice for your child.

THURSDAY

ENTRÉE (choice of one)

- ⅔ cup spaghetti with marinara sauce (2 **Greens**)
- ½ cup spaghetti with meat sauce (**Yellow**)
- Barbecue ribs on wheat bun: 3 ribs (**Red**) and wheat bun (**Yellow**)

SIDES (choice of one)

- Green peas, salad with spinach, apple (**Free Fuel**); 1 tablespoon dressing (**Green**)
- Fruit salad: orange and kiwi, ½ cup pineapple (**Free Fuel**)
- Applesauce: ½ cup (**Green**)

FRIDAY

ENTRÉE (choice of one)

- Chicken nuggets with brown rice: 3 nuggets (**Yellow**) and ½ cup brown rice (**Green**)
- Cheese quesadilla: ½ quesadilla (**Yellow**)

- Hamburger on wheat bun: hamburger and wheat bun (**Red**), and 1 slice cheese (**Green**)

SIDES (choice of one)

- Potato rounds: ¾ cup (**Yellow**)
- Soup: 1 cup (**Green**)
- Mixed vegetables, broccoli, carrot slims, ½ cup pineapple, 1 cup cantaloupe and strawberries (**Free Fuel**)

BYOL: A Wheat, a Meat, and a Treat!

A helpful way to think about creating a wholesome lunch for your child is to pick a wheat, a meat, and a treat, plus a **Free Fuel.** This means whole grain bread; a serving of lean meat; a **Green Light** treat such as fig bars, oatmeal cookies, or graham crackers; and a piece of fruit or some fresh veggies. This balanced lunch will provide your child with a variety of nutrients, including fiber, calcium, protein, and iron.

Here are a few ideas for how you can create a healthy lunch assembly line in your kitchen.

PICK A WHEAT

2 slices reduced-calorie bread
1 light English muffin
1 small pita
2 slices thinly sliced rye bread
1 light hamburger roll
1 6-inch wheat tortilla

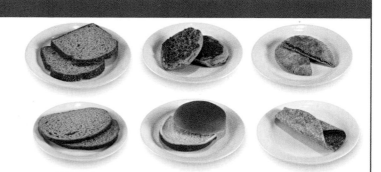

PICK A MEAT

6 slices turkey breast lunch meat
4 slices ham
4 slices roast beef
2 ounces grilled chicken breast
5 slices fat-free bologna
1 tablespoon peanut butter (± sugar-free jelly)

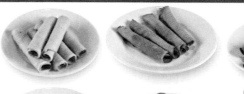

PICK A TREAT

100-calorie pack of anything
20 small pretzel twists
10 baked potato chips
2 small reduced-fat cookies
Quaker low-calorie granola bar

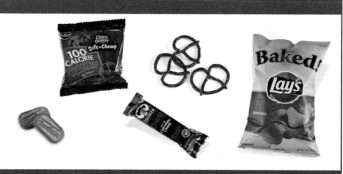

Don't forget to include FREE FUEL in the form of a fruit or veggie, along with a beverage such as water.

What's for Lunch?

It's surprisingly easy to pack a healthy lunch for your kids. Here are 14 sample menus to get you started. Remember to select foods that fit into your child's personalized meal plan.

OPTION 1

6 slices deli turkey meat (**Green**)

2 slices fat-free American cheese (**Free Fuel**)

2 slices reduced-calorie bread (**Green**)

Sliced red bell pepper, cherry tomatoes, celery sticks, or baby carrots (**Free Fuel**)

1 HEALTHY CHOCOLATE CHIP COOKIE (page 88) (**Green**)

OPTION 2

1 serving CREAM OF VEGETABLE SOUP (page 63) (**Green**)

Tuna sandwich: ½ can tuna (canned in water) (**Green**)

3 tablespoons fat-free mayo (**Free Fuel**)

2 slices reduced-calorie bread (**Green**)

OPTION 3

5 slices fat-free bologna (**Green**)

1 slice fat-free cheese (**Free Fuel**)

2 slices reduced-calorie bread (**Green**)

2 pretzel rods (**Green**)

1 cup of grapes (**Free Fuel**)

OPTION 4

2 (97 percent) fat-free hot dogs (**Green**)

1 light hot dog bun (**Green**)

Sauerkraut (**Free Fuel**)

100-calorie pack of cookies (**Green**)

1 pickle (**Free Fuel**)

OPTION 5

1 small slice PERFECT PARTY PIZZA (page 74) (**Yellow**)

Side salad with 1 tablespoon fat-free Italian dressing (**Free Fuel**)

1 PEANUT BUTTER COOKIE (page 87) (**Green**)

OPTION 6

Peanut butter and jelly sandwich: 1 tablespoon peanut butter (**Green**)

1 tablespoon sugar-free jelly (**Free Fuel**)

2 slices reduced-calorie bread (**Green**)

1 banana, sliced (**Free Fuel**)

11 SunChips (**Green**)

OPTION 7

4 slices roast beef lunch meat (**Green**)

2 slices reduced-calorie bread (**Green**)

20 small pretzel twists (**Green**)

Cucumber slices (**Free Fuel**)

OPTION 8

1 BLACK BEAN BURGER (page 77) (**Yellow**)

1 light hamburger bun (**Green**)

1 pickle (**Free Fuel**)

1 medium orange (**Free Fuel**)

OPTION 9

Leftover OVEN-FRIED CHICKEN (page 78) (**Green, Green**)

Store-bought cucumber sushi roll (without avocado), prepared with brown rice (**Green + Free Fuel**)

OPTION 10

1 CRUSTLESS MINIQUICHE (page 80) (**Green**)

1 cup POTATO SALAD (page 82) (**Yellow**)

1 medium banana (**Free Fuel**)

OPTION 11

1 6-inch Roasted Chicken Breast Sub from Subway (no cheese or mayo) (**Yellow + Green**)

2 clementines (**Free Fuel**)

OPTION 12

½ cup CHICKEN SALAD (page 81) (**Green**)

2 slices rye bread, thinly sliced (**Green**)

Lettuce and tomato (**Free Fuel**)

¾ cup chicken noodle soup (**Green**)

OPTION 13

1 cup TURKEY AND BLACK BEAN CHILI (page 84) (**Yellow + Green**)

1 medium apple (**Free Fuel**)

OPTION 14

1 reduced-calorie English muffin (**Green**)

1 tablespoon almond butter (**Green**)

3 tablespoons sugar-free jelly (**Free Fuel**)

100-calorie pack Doritos (**Green**)

1 medium peach (**Free Fuel**)

Grade-A Lunch Recipes

Most of these yummy lunches can be easily wrapped up and packed in a lunch box, and some—such as the Turkey and Black Bean Chili (page 84)—are perfect for hearty weekend lunches with the whole family. There's something here to please everyone's taste buds!

Perfect Party Pizza

Get the whole family involved in making this delicious pizza. Using fat-free cheese is a great way to trim fat and calories from your favorite recipes.

MAKES 8 SERVINGS ■ EACH SERVING (1 SLICE, OR ¼ PIE) = 1 YELLOW

PREP TIME: 10 minutes
COOK TIME: 10 minutes
READY TIME: 20 minutes

1 package Italian-style
    spaghetti sauce mix
1 teaspoon oregano leaves
⅛ teaspoon crushed red pepper
    (optional)
1¼ cups tomato puree
¼ cup water
2 (12-inch) whole wheat pizza
    crusts
2 cups shredded fat-free
    mozzarella cheese

1. Preheat the oven to 400°F.

2. Combine the spaghetti sauce mix, oregano leaves, red pepper if using, tomato puree, and water in a bowl.

3. Spread the mixture over each pizza crust to within 1 inch of the edge.

4. Sprinkle each pizza crust with the mozzarella cheese and other healthy pizza toppings, if desired.

5. Bake in the oven for 10 minutes or until the crust is crisp and the cheese is melted.

6. Cut each pizza into 4 slices; place 1 slice on a plate and serve immediately.

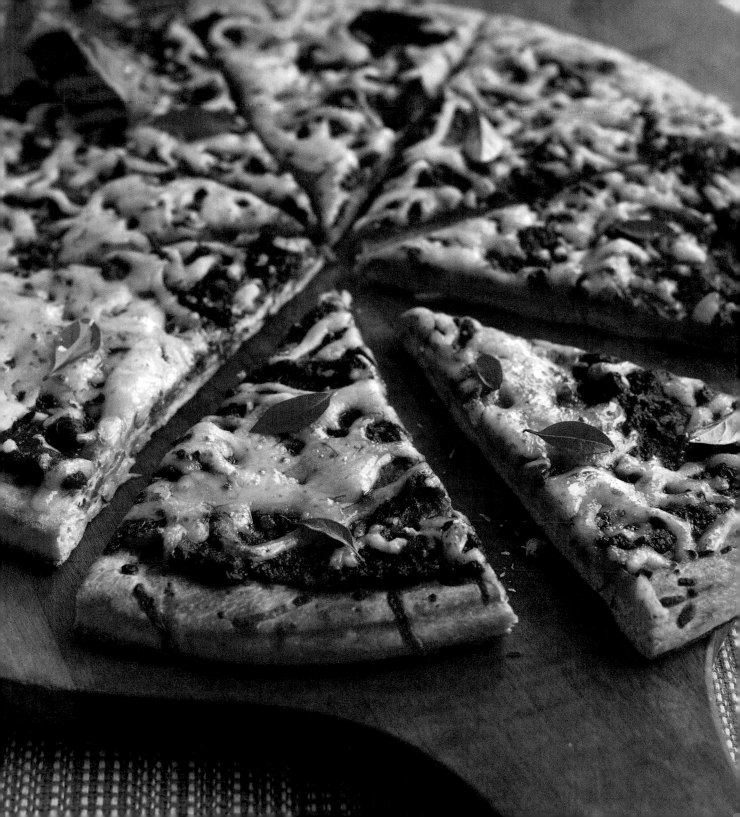

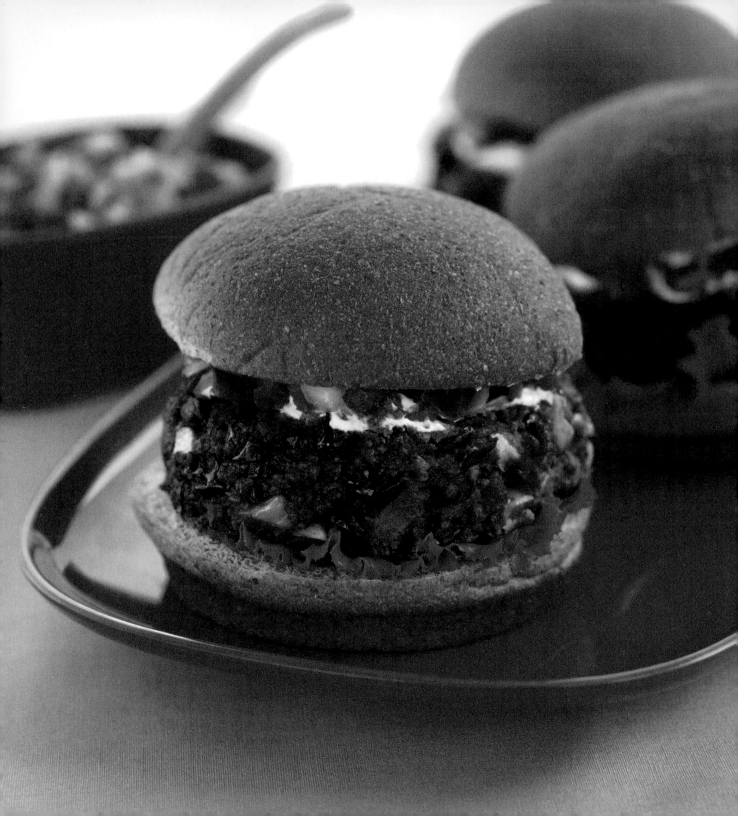

Black Bean Burgers

Black Bean Burgers make a great alternative to beef burgers. These burgers cook very well in a hot oven or in a nonstick skillet for 3 to 4 minutes per side. Serve on a whole grain bun with fat-free sour cream and plenty of salsa. They're perfect for weekend lunches.

MAKES 4 BURGERS ■ EACH SERVING (1 BURGER) = 1 YELLOW ;
1 LIGHT WHOLE WHEAT BUN = 1 GREEN ●; ½ CUP FAT-FREE SOUR CREAM = 1 GREEN ●

PREP TIME: 15 minutes

COOK TIME: 15 minutes

READY TIME: 30 minutes

Vegetable cooking spray

1 (15-ounce) can low-sodium black beans, drained

½ cup dry bread crumbs

⅓–½ cup finely chopped onion

⅓ cup tomato sauce

1 teaspoon cumin

2 tablespoons chopped cilantro

½ cup fat-free sour cream

½ cup salsa

1. Preheat the oven to 400°F and coat a baking sheet with cooking spray.

2. In a medium bowl, mash the beans with a fork or potato masher.

3. Add the bread crumbs, onion, tomato sauce, cumin, and cilantro.

4. Blend with a fork.

5. Form into 4 patties and place on the baking sheet.

6. Bake for 15 minutes.

7. Remove carefully with a spatula and place on a bun. Top with lettuce, tomato, sour cream, or salsa, as desired.

Oven-Fried Chicken

This satisfying recipe tastes even better than deep-fried chicken and is wonderful hot or cold. It's perfect to pack in lunch boxes!

MAKES 4 SERVINGS ■ EACH SERVING (2 PIECES) = 2 GREENS

PREP TIME: 20 minutes
COOK TIME: 40–50 minutes
READY TIME: 1 hour–1 hour 10 minutes

½ cup buttermilk

1 tablespoon Dijon mustard

2 garlic cloves, minced

1 teaspoon hot sauce

2½–3 pounds chicken thighs and drumsticks, skin removed

Vegetable cooking spray

½ cup whole wheat flour

1½ tablespoons sesame seeds

1½ teaspoons paprika

1 teaspoon dried thyme leaves

1 teaspoon baking powder

¼ teaspoon salt

¼ teaspoon ground black pepper

Olive oil cooking spray

4 cups frozen green beans

1. Whisk the buttermilk, mustard, garlic, and hot sauce in a small bowl until well blended.

2. Add the chicken pieces and turn to coat.

3. Cover the bowl and marinate the chicken in the refrigerator for at least ½ hour or for up to 8 hours.

4. Preheat the oven to 425°F. Line a baking sheet with foil. Set a wire rack on the baking sheet and coat it with vegetable cooking spray.

5. Whisk the flour, sesame seeds, paprika, thyme, baking powder, salt, and pepper in a small bowl.

6. Place the flour mixture in a large sealable plastic bag. Working with 1 or 2 pieces of chicken at a time, shake off the excess marinade and place the chicken in the bag. Shake to coat. Remove the chicken, shake off the excess flour, and place the chicken on the prepared rack.

7. Spray the chicken pieces with olive oil cooking spray.

8. Bake the chicken until golden brown and no longer pink in the center, 40 to 50 minutes.

9. Prepare the green beans according to the package directions and serve with the chicken.

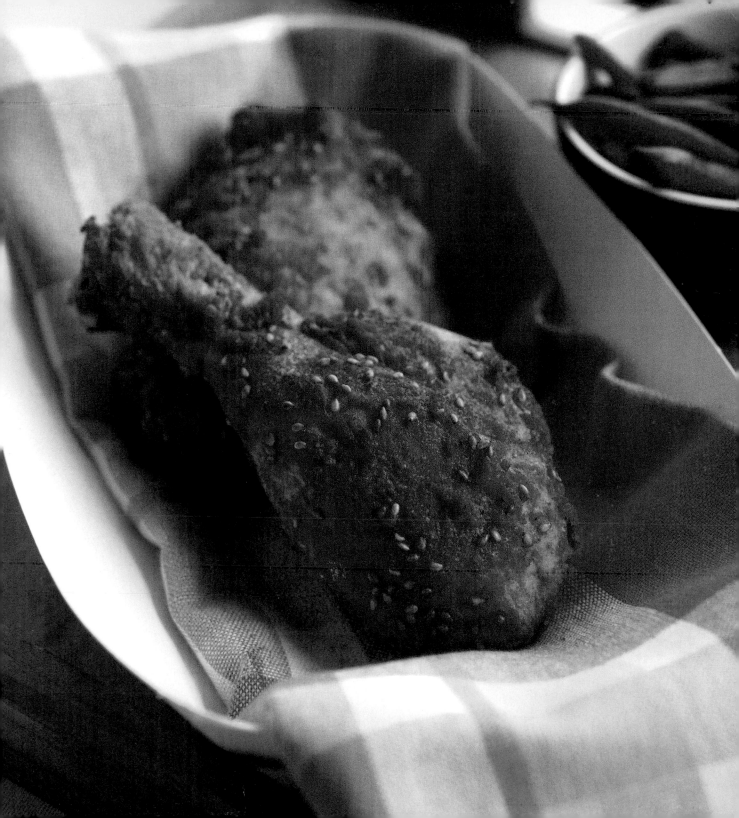

Crustless Miniquiches

Who says quiche needs a crust? This recipe certainly doesn't. It's a great example of how you can make any recipe healthier by using nutritious substitutions. You can freeze these miniquiches in zip-top bags and then reheat on a cookie sheet.

MAKES 24 MINIQUICHES ■ EACH SERVING (1 MINIQUICHE) = 1 GREEN

PREP TIME: 10 minutes

COOK TIME: 10–12 minutes

READY TIME: 30 minutes

3 (6-ounce) containers fat-free
    feta cheese

⅓ cup flour

1 teaspoon baking powder

20 ounces frozen spinach,
    thawed and squeezed dry

20 egg whites

⅔ cup fat-free milk

Vegetable cooking spray

1. Preheat the oven to 350°F.

2. In a large bowl, mix the cheese, flour, baking powder, and spinach.

3. In a separate bowl, whisk together the egg whites and milk.

4. Pour the egg white mixture onto the spinach mixture and gently fold together.

5. Lightly spray nonstick muffin pans with cooking spray.

6. Fill each muffin cup about three-quarters full with the quiche mixture.

7. Bake for 20 to 22 minutes or until set.

8. Carefully loosen and remove the quiches from the muffin tins. Cool on a cooling rack for a few minutes and serve.

Chicken Salad

I always suggest to the families I work with that they use fat-free mayonnaise in traditional recipes like this one. No one will be able to tell the difference, but the savings in calories and fat are well worth the switch.

MAKES 4 SERVINGS ■ EACH SERVING (½ CUP) = 1 GREEN

PREP TIME: 15 minutes

COOK TIME: 5–10 minutes

READY TIME: 40 minutes

Vegetable cooking spray

8 ounces chicken breast chunks

3 tablespoons fat-free mayonnaise

⅓ cup green seedless grapes, halved

½ green apple, chopped

1. In a pan coated with cooking spray, sauté the chicken until it is fully cooked, approximately 5 to 10 minutes.

2. Let cool 15 minutes.

3. Mix all ingredients together.

Potato Salad

We all know tofu is healthy—but how can you get your kids to embrace it? Here's a solution your family will love.

MAKES 8 SERVINGS ■ EACH SERVING (1 CUP) = 1 YELLOW

PREP TIME: 10 minutes
COOK TIME: 20–25 minutes
READY TIME: 4½ hours

3 pounds round red potatoes

12 ounces soft silken-style tofu

3 tablespoons lemon juice

1 teaspoon mustard

1 garlic clove, minced

1 teaspoon salt

1 teaspoon ground black pepper

2 tablespoons olive oil

3 hard-boiled eggs

½ cup chopped celery

1 medium red bell pepper, chopped

⅓ cup chopped scallions

½ cup chopped dill pickles

1. Place the potatoes in a covered pot with lightly salted water. Bring to a boil, reduce the heat, and simmer for 20 to 25 minutes until the potatoes are tender. Drain, peel, and cube the potatoes.

2. In a blender or food processor, combine the tofu, lemon juice, mustard, garlic, salt, and pepper. Process until smooth. Add the oil slowly and steadily.

3. Peel and roughly chop the eggs.

4. In a large bowl, combine the eggs, potatoes, celery, bell pepper, scallions, and pickles. Add the tofu dressing, tossing lightly. Season to taste with additional salt and pepper.

5. Cover and chill for at least 4 hours.

6. To enhance freshness before serving, stir in 1 tablespoon milk or pickle juice.

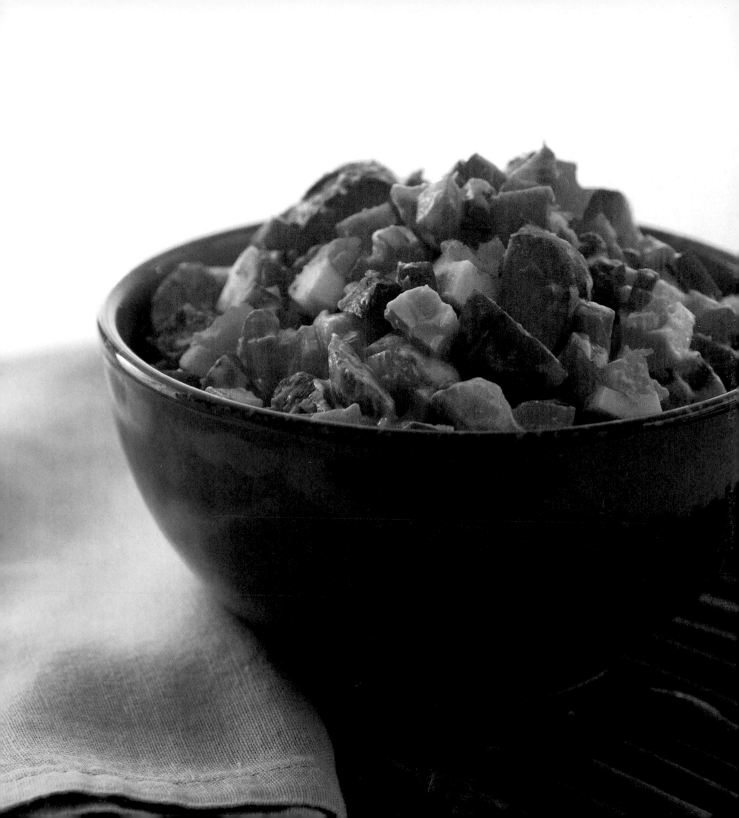

Turkey and Black Bean Chili

Black beans have a meaty flavor all their own. Add in ground turkey or "vegetarian ground meat" (found in the frozen foods aisle) and serve with a side of green salad, and you've got a hearty lunch sure to satisfy every member of the family.

MAKES 6 SERVINGS ■ EACH SERVING (1 CUP) = 1 YELLOW ● + 1 GREEN ●
EACH SERVING (1 CUP) VEGETARIAN SUBSTITUTE = 1 YELLOW ●

PREP TIME: 10 minutes
COOK TIME: 10–15 minutes
READY TIME: 25 minutes

1 tablespoon olive oil

½ medium yellow onion, diced (about 1 cup)

1 teaspoon minced garlic (about 2 cloves)

1 pound ground turkey or vegetarian ground meat

1 tablespoon chili powder

15 ounces diced tomatoes with green chile peppers

6 ounces tomato paste

9–10 ounces naturally sweetened canned corn, drained

15 ounces canned black beans, drained and rinsed

Dash of hot pepper sauce (such as Tabasco)

1. In a stockpot, heat the oil over medium heat.

2. Add the onion and cook until tender, about 3 minutes.

3. Add the garlic and stir for about 30 seconds, then add the turkey and chili powder and brown the turkey for about 5 minutes, until it is mostly cooked through. (If you are using vegetarian "meat," add it to the pot in step 4, as there is no need to brown it.)

4. Add the diced tomatoes, tomato paste, corn, and beans, and bring to a simmer.

5. Simmer the chili for 10 to 15 minutes, stirring occasionally.

6. Spoon into individual bowls and serve with a dash of hot pepper sauce.

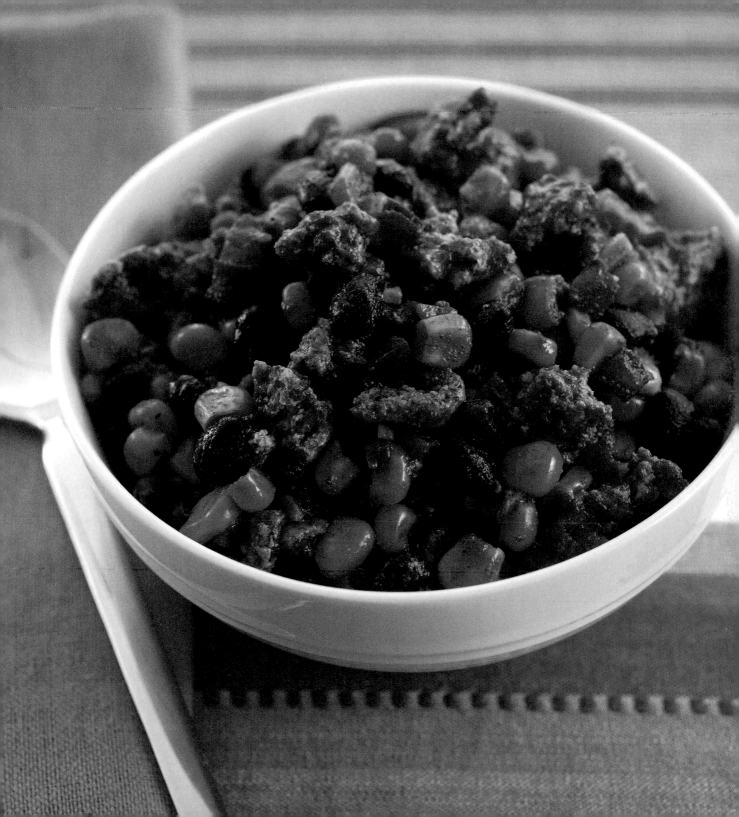

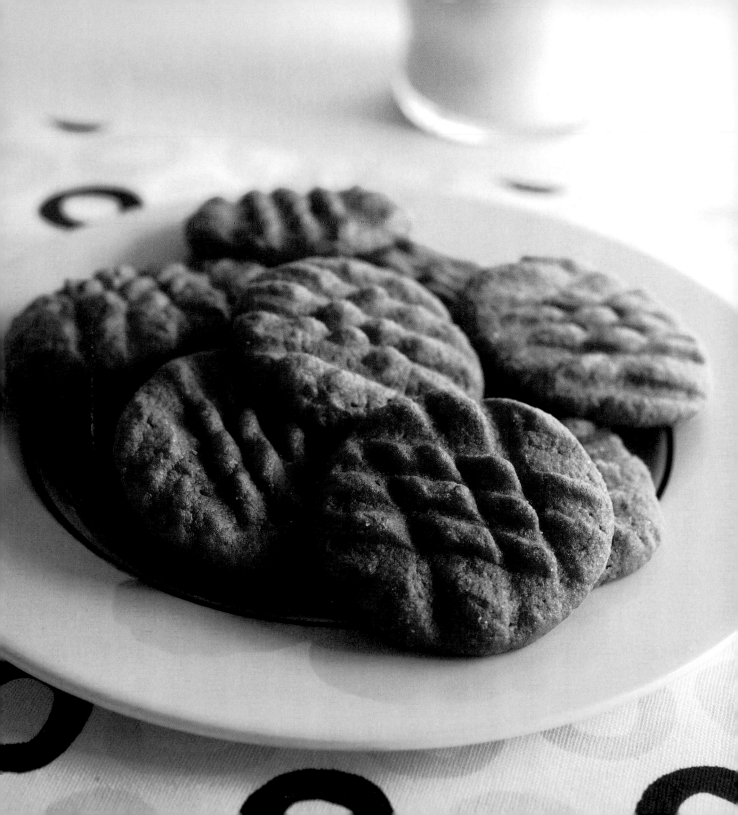

Peanut Butter Cookies

The whole wheat flour used in these yummy cookies increases the fiber and nutrition content, and the peanut butter contributes a protein punch. My kids love cookies as their lunch "treat."

MAKES 36 COOKIES ■ EACH SERVING (1 COOKIE) = 1 GREEN

PREP TIME: 20 minutes
COOK TIME: 15 minutes
READY TIME: 35 minutes

1 cup creamy peanut butter
½ cup butter, softened
½ cup honey
½ cup packed brown sugar
1 egg
1½ cups whole wheat flour
1 teaspoon baking powder

1. Preheat the oven to 350°F.

2. In a large bowl, mix the peanut butter, butter, honey, sugar, and egg until smooth.

3. Combine the flour and baking powder.

4. Stir the flour mixture into the peanut butter batter until blended.

5. Roll the dough into small balls and place on greased baking sheets.

6. Flatten each ball slightly with a fork.

7. Bake for 13 to 15 minutes or until the cookies are slightly toasted at the edges.

8. Cool on cooling rack.

Healthy Chocolate Chip Cookies

What kid can go without chocolate chip cookies? Here's a healthier version of this classic treat. It has all the flavor of—but less fat than—a regular chocolate chip cookie.

MAKES 36 COOKIES ■ EACH SERVING (1 COOKIE) = 1 GREEN

PREP TIME: 8 minutes
COOK TIME: 12–14 minutes
READY TIME: 30 minutes

1 cup whole wheat flour

1 cup oat flour

2 teaspoons baking powder

¾ teaspoon salt

¼ teaspoon ground nutmeg

¼ teaspoon ground cinnamon

½ cup butter, softened

¾ cup brown sugar

1 egg

¼ cup fat-free milk

5 ounces bittersweet chocolate chips

1. Preheat the oven to 350°F.

2. In a medium bowl, stir together the flours, baking powder, salt, nutmeg, and cinnamon.

3. In a large mixing bowl, cream the butter and sugar together until light and fluffy.

4. Beat the egg into the butter mixture, then beat in the milk.

5. Stir in the flour mixture.

6. Stir in the chocolate chips.

7. Drop the dough by rounded teaspoons onto greased cookie sheets.

8. Bake for 12 to 14 minutes or until the cookies are browned around the edges.

9. Transfer to a cooling rack and cool for 10 minutes before serving.

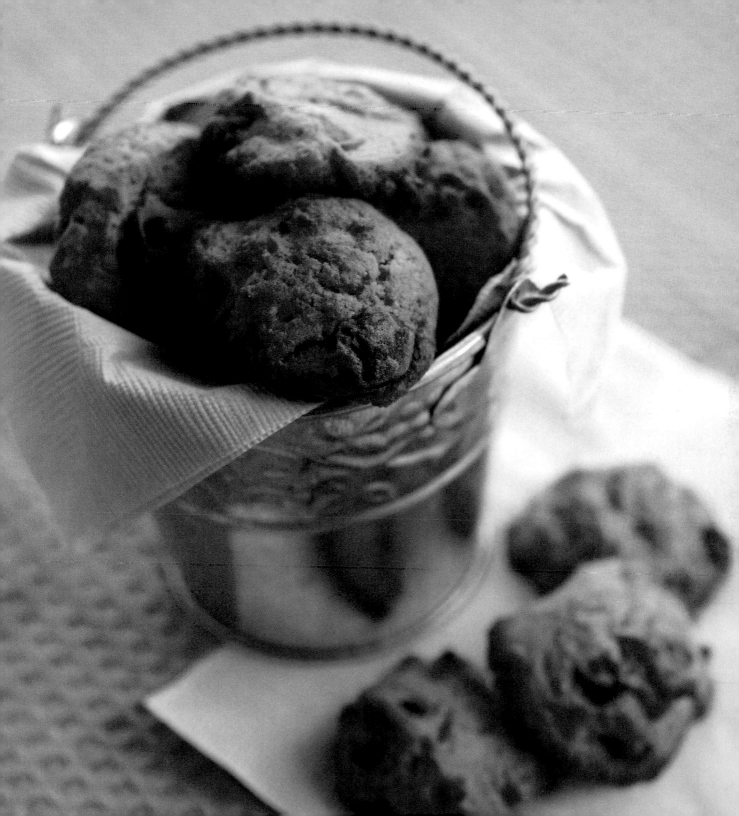

Green Light Sandwich Alternatives

If your child's lunch box is always filled with the same boring sandwich, he's probably trading it to a classmate for a less-healthy option. It's time to step on the gas and change lanes! With just a little effort and creativity, you can create packed lunches your child will love—not barter for chips. Here are some ideas to inspire you.

● Make homemade "lunchables." Pack whole grain crackers; low-fat or fat-free cheese; a serving of lean turkey, chicken, ham, or roast beef; and some veggie sticks and let your child assemble his or her own lunch.

● Pack a serving of tuna salad (made with fat-free mayo) as a dip for whole wheat crackers, carrot sticks, and cucumber slices.

● Mash up a serving of avocado and add a little lime juice so it doesn't turn brown. Pack it as a dip with veggies or whole wheat crackers.

● For sandwiches, experiment with different breads, including whole wheat, rye, pita pockets, English muffins, or even minibagels. Higher-fiber breads will keep your kids feeling fuller longer.

● Try substituting almond butter or another nut butter for peanut butter in their regular PB&J sandwich. You can experiment with different flavors of sugar-free jams and jellies, as well.

● For younger kids, try using cookie cutters in the form of hearts, stars, or flowers to cut sandwiches into fun shapes. Let them choose the cookie cutter they want and help you press out the shapes!

● Make variations of their favorite combinations—try sandwiches made with peanut butter and a sliced banana, lean turkey with hummus, or low-fat or fat-free cream cheese with sugar-free jelly or jam.

● Consider substituting lettuce for bread and making lettuce wraps with meat and cheese.

● If your child loves sweet, spicy flavors, try spreading apple butter on a slice of whole grain bread. Top it with fresh apple slices, raisins, and a sprinkle of cinnamon.

● In a small Thermos, pack a serving of pasta salad made with whole wheat pasta, fat-free dressing, and chopped veggies like bell peppers and cherry tomatoes.

FROM RED LIGHT TO GREEN LIGHT: LUNCH MAKEOVERS

With some easy substitutions, you can cut down on a recipe's fat, calories, and cholesterol—without reducing the flavor. Here's how to turn **Red Light** pit stops into **Green Light** lunches.

HIGH-CALORIE RED LIGHT FOODS	LOW-CALORIE GREEN LIGHT FOODS	
Grilled cheese sandwich	Place 3 slices fat-free American cheese between 2 slices reduced-calorie bread and toast in the toaster oven until the cheese has melted.	●
Tuna salad sandwich	Make tuna salad made with ½ can drained, canned tuna (packed in water) mixed with 2 tablespoons fat-free mayonnaise and served on 2 slices reduced-calorie bread.	●●
Pizza bagel	Cut a medium-size bagel in half and toast 1 half. Then top with ½ cup marinara sauce and ¼ cup fat-free mozzarella cheese and place under the broiler until the cheese is melted.	●●
Chicken nuggets	Bake 6 frozen chicken nuggets in the oven on a cookie sheet.	●●●
Macaroni and cheese	Cook 1 cup whole wheat elbow macaroni and stir in 2 slices fat-free American cheese while the pasta is still steaming hot.	●●●
BLT	Combine 2 slices reduced-calorie whole wheat bread, toasted, with 2 slices cooked turkey bacon, lettuce, tomato, and fat-free mayonnaise.	●●
Steak sandwich on a hard roll	Assemble a sandwich with 3 ounces lean sirloin steak and onions sautéed in fat-free cooking spray on 2 slices light whole wheat bread.	●●
Bowl of New England clam chowder	Prepare 1 cup canned New England clam chowder using fat-free milk.	●●

BYOL Time-Savers

With kids getting ready for school and Mom and Dad hurrying off to work, weekday mornings are often hectic. It's tough enough to get breakfast on the table, let alone find time to pack healthy lunches for the day ahead. But with just a little planning and preparation, you can overcome this challenge. A good example is Meredith, age 12, who told me she couldn't bring lunch because she didn't have time to pack it. We went through her schedule, and I gave her two choices: Make lunch the night before or get up 15 minutes earlier in the morning. Not surprisingly, she chose the night before.

To keep her sandwich from getting soggy, Meredith wrapped each component in its own zip-top bag so she could assemble it at lunchtime. She even got a tiny reusable container for her fat-free mayonnaise so she could spread it on the bread at lunch. Meredith later told me that it was easier to make five of these disassembled sandwiches on Sunday night and grab one each morning. She got out of the house faster in the morning and enjoyed her food. And she lost weight!

Always remember that it's important to follow food safety precautions when you pack your child's lunch. Don't include foods that contain raw eggs or fish, like refrigerated cookie dough or sushi. Foods that require refrigeration (such as meat and dairy products like yogurt) should not be left unrefrigerated for more than 2 hours. Use a well-insulated lunch box and include an ice pack or a frozen water bottle to keep such foods cold until lunchtime. Go-Gurts are a great choice for school lunches because they can go straight from the freezer to the lunch bag and will defrost in time for lunch.

When it comes to our children, the quality of nourishment we provide for their growing bodies and minds will influence the people they later become. Letting them eat junky cafeteria food is easy and might be tempting at times. But as parents, we have a responsibility to give our kids the nutrients they need. It's important to put our families' health first and to ensure our kids are given the wholesome foods they require for a healthy, active life.

6

● ● ●

AFTERNOON SNACK ATTACKS

I'm constantly on the lookout for new snacks for my children, because what they love one week they might get bored with the next. For afternoon snacks, my kids love low-fat cheese sticks (**Green**); apple slices (**Free Fuel**) with a tablespoon of peanut butter (**Green**); 100-calorie packs (**Green**); any type of fruit (**Free Fuel**); pistachio nuts (**Green**); and my personal favorite: fat-free frozen yogurt (4 ounces is a **Green**). I'm addicted to cappuccino flavor, and I eat it every single day for *my* snack!

For more "junky" **Green Light** snacks, we make a healthier version of s'mores at home. We break one graham cracker (**Green**) in half and put two gooey marshmallows (**Green**) on each half. We usually do this in our backyard, roasting the marshmallows in our fire pit. The kids love to hunt for sticks to use to roast the marshmallows. But if you don't want to build a fire (or if the weather doesn't cooperate), you could also melt the marshmallows in the microwave. Leaving out the chocolate saves a **Yellow Light,** and the kids usually don't notice the difference.

Just because my kids have learned to eat healthy snacks doesn't mean we haven't experienced a few temper tantrums along the way. Together with some of the other moms from my kids' school, we used to take our kids to a café after school every day, and most of the other moms let their children eat sweets there. I found myself in a predicament. I didn't want my children to eat chocolate every day, but it seemed unfair for them to sit there and watch the other kids eat candy bars. My other option was to avoid the café and have my kids miss out on the fun. Should I isolate my kids just to keep them healthy? I decided on a compromise. I explained to my children that chocolate is not a healthy every-day snack. "Some days, you can go to the café and have chocolate, but most days you have to pick from the healthy snacks, like the granola bars or pretzels," I told them.

At first, this solution was met with screams and tears. But eventually, they learned that we have special days for treats. When situations like this arise with my children, I simply say, "Different mommies have different rules." Eventually, my children sat and ate their pretzels happily, while their friends ate chocolate. They didn't cry, complain, or beg me for candy. They realized that the fun was in being with their friends, not in eating a treat. You would be surprised by how quickly kids can adapt to any situation if you just hang in there. (I was later able to convince the café to serve more healthy snack options, as well, like fresh fruit and yogurt!)

The Super Nutrient for Afternoon Snacks

Children's tummies are small, but their energy needs are large. In the afternoon, kids often want empty carbohydrates that give them an immediate sugar spike, like candy bars, cookies, and other sugary snacks. The best way for them to get energy is not through sugary foods but through complex carbs, which supply fiber. Fiber is the part of fruits, vegetables, beans, and grains that the body can't break down—like the skins of fruits and vegetables. Fiber is never absorbed into the bloodstream. Instead, it moves through the intestines, giving a feeling of fullness while providing few calories. When afternoon snacks incorporate fiber, a child's energy burst lasts until dinner.

So, when planning afternoon snacks for your kids, you'll want to include snack foods with ample fiber. For example:

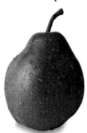

● **Fruit such as apples, pears, and berries.** These foods are loaded not only with fiber but also with antioxidants, which help your children stay healthy.

● **Vegetables—all kinds.** These foods make super snacks! Two whole carrots, for example, have 3 grams of fiber. Plus, vegetables are low in calories, so your kids can fill up on lots of them every day.

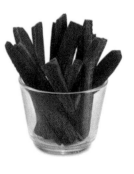

The Scoop on Sugar and Sugar Substitutes

Parents often ask me if they should allow their kids to eat sugar. It's certainly true that eating too many sugary foods can contribute to obesity and promote tooth decay, so it's best to limit your child's sugar intake. The problem, however, is that sugar is added to many foods, from soft drinks and candy to cereals and snack foods. When you read the labels of these products, keep in mind that sugar is often hidden under different names: Corn syrup or sweetener, fruit juice concentrate, dextrose, fructose, honey, and molasses are all forms of sugar.

One of the most widely used sweeteners in packaged foods is high fructose corn syrup (HFCS), which is also a preservative. Because it extends the shelf life of foods and is cheaper than sugar, HFCS has become a popular ingredient in many sodas, fruit-flavored drinks, and other processed foods.

HFCS in itself does not increase the risk of obesity. Obesity is caused by taking in more calories than are burned. But many foods containing HFCS are loaded with calories. Therefore, if your children eat a lot of these foods, they will gain weight. There is no nutritional difference between HFCS and sugar. Both contain the same number of calories. All forms of sugar will cause weight gain if eaten in excess.

If you are concerned about the amount of sugar in your family's diet, consider these tips:

- Limit the processed foods you keep in the house.

- Avoid foods that contain a large amount of added sugar in any form.

- Avoid soda, juice, and other sweetened beverages.

- Use artificial sweeteners, in moderation. I prefer Splenda (sucralose), made from a process that starts with sugar. It may be safely used by everyone, including children.

- If you dislike the idea of using artificial sweeteners but want to avoid sugar, try a natural sweetener such as agave nectar, which is a plant extract. It contains only 2.9 calories per gram compared to sugar's 4, and because it's sweeter than sugar, you need less. You can bake with agave nectar. Another natural sweetener worth trying is stevia (Truvia). It is calorie free and up to 300 times sweeter than sugar. I don't recommend baking with stevia, however.

- Old favorites such as honey, maple syrup, brown rice syrup, sorghum, and molasses contain about as many calories as sugar, but also contain natural antioxidants, vitamins, and other nutrients.

- For baking, try using the natural sugars in fruit to sweeten your food, such as mashed bananas, pureed figs, or applesauce.

- **Nuts.** These crunchy treats are rich in monounsaturated fat, which is good for heart and muscle health.

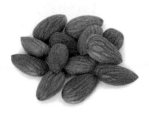

- **Popcorn.** For fiber, nothing beats air-popped popcorn as a snack. One serving of popcorn gives a child six times more fiber than one serving of potato chips. That's because popcorn supplies whole corn kernels and is thus a whole grain. Most potato chips are refined; they're peeled, for example, and that removes most of the fiber. Popcorn makes for a great low-calorie snack because 3 whole cups (a big bowl) is a **Green** serving. That's a big snack! When buying microwave popcorn, remember to choose the 94 percent fat-free popcorn to maximize the health benefits.

- **Flax.** Add some ground flaxseed to your meals, in soups, casseroles, smoothies, or salads. Flaxseed is an excellent source of omega-3 fatty acids, which have been linked to a lower risk of heart disease. One ounce, which is about 3 tablespoons, contains 7 grams of fiber.

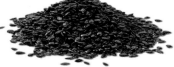

Backpack Snacks

Do your children go straight from school to afternoon activities? If so, they'll usually be ravenous, so you'll want to pack **Green Light** snacks that are easily transportable in snack-size zip-top bags or resealable containers. If you give kids the exact portion size, they won't be tempted to overeat. Great "backpackable" **Green Light** snacks include:

- 3 cups air-popped or 94 percent fat-free microwave popcorn
- Cut-up raw vegetables and ¼ cup hummus
- Low-fat string cheese
- Soft granola bar
- 1 tablespoon peanut butter and apple slices (Put lemon juice on the apple slices so they don't brown, or buy the prepackaged slices.)
- 2 tablespoons trail mix
- ¾ cup dry breakfast cereal (high fiber, low sugar)
- Higher-fiber, lower-fat crackers (Serving size varies based on brand.)

Admittedly, there will be days when you don't have time to fix afternoon snacks, and you'll give your child some money to purchase a snack instead. Be careful here! An older patient of mine, 15-year-old Eddie, used to stop at the deli on his way home from school each day. He would buy a soda and some chips. His mother felt that she couldn't control this habit because she wasn't there.

I told her that communication was the key. She should first let Eddie know that she would not give him money if he was going to use it to buy junk. Then we brainstormed some healthier options. I suggested that Eddie buy flavored seltzer water rather than regular sodas. Soft drinks are a big problem for kids of all ages. The American Academy of Pediatrics cites the high volume of sugar in those drinks as a leading cause of obesity in children. Choosing flavored seltzer water over soda just once a day would cut about 150 calories (or a **Yellow Light** serving) from Eddie's diet!

Eddie didn't want to give up the chips, so we compromised. Instead of buying a two-serving-size bag of greasy chips at the deli, his mom put a serving of baked chips in his backpack each day. As an extra incentive, Eddie and his mother banked the money he was saving by eating the baked chips from home and kept it in a special bowl. Mom then agreed to match the money in the bowl to help Eddie purchase something special that he really wanted. In just a few months, he saved enough money to buy an iPod—and lost weight in the process.

Home after School? Play the Snack Game!

What if your kids come straight home after school? If you or another adult is there to supervise them, try to make the afternoon snack a fun experience. Younger kids love to play with their food. You can turn a healthy snack into a game by encouraging this "bad" habit. Allow your children to participate in snack preparation and let them have fun eating. Serve snacks in unusual containers. Place snacks on the plate in interesting shapes. Or experiment with different methods, textures, and mouth feels. The following action verbs make snacktime fun.

Dipping

- Cut apples into small pieces and put them on toothpicks. Dip the pieces into melted fat-free cheese (**Free Fuel**) or 4 ounces fat-free flavored yogurt (**Green**).
- Dip 12 baked tortilla chips (**Green**) in salsa (**Free Fuel**).
- Make an apple fondue. Melt 1 tablespoon peanut butter (**Green**) in a bowl. Cut an apple (**Free Fuel**) into wedges and let your children dip the wedges into the peanut butter.
- Create a cheese fondue. Melt ½ cup shredded low-fat cheese (**Green**) in a bowl. Cut veggies (**Free**

Fuel) into small sticks and let children dip them into the cheese.

- Dip 4 pieces of pita into ¼ cup GARLIC AND SUN-DRIED TOMATO HUMMUS (page 101) (**Yellow**).

Freezing

- Freeze grapes or bananas (both **Free Fuel**) for a refreshing snack.
- Serve frozen fruit bars (**Yellow**) for afternoon snacks—or make your own ice pops. Try the FROZEN YOGURT POPS (page 104) (**Green**).

Blending

- Whip up some homemade smoothies: Blend 1 cup fat-free milk, 3 ice cubes, and fruit in a blender. Add a dash of vanilla, cinnamon, or nutmeg for extra flavor (**Green**).
- Make a banana shake: Place half of a frozen banana in a blender, add fat-free milk, and puree until creamy (**Green**). This is one of my favorites!

Spearing

- Give your kids wooden skewers so they can spear pieces of fruit: apples, bananas, grapes, pears, peaches, strawberries, plums, honeydew, cantaloupe, watermelon, pineapple, kiwis, blackberries, blueberries, raspberries, apricots, mangos, figs, tangerines, guavas, or star fruit (**Free Fuel**).
- Create FUN FRUIT KEBOBS (page 103). Two skewers equals one **Green Light** food.

Melting

- Place a slice of fat-free cheese (**Free Fuel**) atop one light English muffin (**Green**). Melt under the broiler or in the toaster oven for a few seconds.
- Make **Green Light** quesadillas: Melt fat-free cheese (**Free Fuel**) on one wheat tortilla (**Green**) or two corn tortillas (**Green**). Top with salsa (**Free Fuel**).
- Create a quick veggie pita pizza: Top a small pita (**Green**) with canned tomato sauce (**Free Fuel**) and fat-free mozzarella cheese (**Free Fuel**). Cover with vegetables (**Green**). Heat in the oven until the cheese melts.

Spreading

- Spread 1 tablespoon peanut butter (**Green**) on 6 reduced-fat Triscuit crackers (**Green**).
- Turn snacks into artwork by making BUGS ON A LOG (page 108) (**Green**).
- Spread ¼ cup hummus (**Green**) on a mini whole wheat pita (**Green**).
- Spread ⅓ cup fat-free cream cheese (**Green**) on celery (**Free Fuel**).

Rolling

- Dip a banana in ⅓ cup low-fat or fat-free yogurt and roll in ¼ cup Rice Krispies (**Green**). Or try BANANA KRISPIE/NUT POPS (page 107) (**Yellow**).
- Slice a banana and coat with cocoa powder (**Free Fuel**). Roll in ½ ounce toasted coconut flakes (**Green**).

Crunching

Kids love to crunch! Play games designed around crunching. Who can crunch carrots the loudest (allowed only at game time), nibble lettuce like a bunny, or pretend to be a giant and munch on broccoli "trees"? All the negative feelings children might have about vegetables disappear when they're having fun with veggies. When they're in the mood for a crunchy snack, here are your best bets.

- An assortment of cut-up fresh veggies (**Free Fuel**)
- 2 flavored rice cakes (**Green**)
- 3 cups 94 percent fat-free microwave popcorn (**Green**)
- Granola bars—less than 100 calories (**Green**)
- Pretzels—2 rods or 20 twists (**Green**)
- 1 full graham cracker (**Green**)
- 10 baked potato chips (**Green**)

- 12 almonds (**Green**)
- ¾ cup nonsugar cereal (most types) with ¼ cup fat-free milk (**Green**)

Spooning

- ½ cup fat-free or low-fat flavored yogurt (**Green**)
- BAKED APPLE (page 111) (**Free Fuel**)
- ⅔ cup fat-free, sugar-free pudding made with fat-free milk (**Green**)
- 1 cup sugar-free Jell-O (**Free Fuel**)
- ¾ cup fat-free cottage cheese (**Green**) and fruit (**Free Fuel**)

Topping

- Top 1 slice reduced-calorie whole wheat bread with 3 slices turkey breast lunch meat (**Green**).
- Top a small (4-ounce) baked potato (**Green**) with salsa (**Free Fuel**) or ½ cup fat-free sour cream (**Green**) or ½ cup fat-free yogurt (**Green**).

Peeling

Peeling uses fingers, and kids love things they can eat with their hands. Here are some suggestions.

- Edamame (**Free Fuel**)
- 1 hard-boiled egg (**Green**)
- Tangerines, clementines, a banana, or any peelable fruit (**Free Fuel**)

What's for an Afternoon Snack?

When planning afternoon snacks for your kids, be sure to include Free Fuel. Here are 14 full snack menus to get you started. Choose foods based on your child's personalized game plan.

SAMPLE SNACKS

OPTION 1

3 cups 94 percent fat-free microwave popcorn (**Green**)

Grapes (**Free Fuel**)

OPTION 2

10 baked potato chips (**Green**)

Salsa (**Free Fuel**)

OPTION 3

1 piece string cheese (**Green**)

1 medium apple (**Free Fuel**)

OPTION 4

10 bagel chips (**Green**)

1 slice fat-free cheese (**Free Fuel**)

Carrot slices (**Free Fuel**)

OPTION 5

100-calorie pack of cookies (**Green**)

1 cup strawberries (**Free Fuel**)

OPTION 6

2 celery stalks (**Free Fuel**)

1 tablespoon peanut butter (**Green**)

OPTION 7

4 ounces fat-free yogurt (**Green**)

Blueberries (**Free Fuel**)

OPTION 8

1 piece string cheese (**Green**)

Sliced red bell peppers (**Free Fuel**)

OPTION 9

20 pistachio nuts (**Green**)

Grapes (**Free Fuel**)

OPTION 10

Carrot and celery sticks (**Free Fuel**)

¼ cup hummus (**Green**)

OPTION 11

2-inch-square Rice Krispies treat (**Green**)

½ cup raspberries (**Free Fuel**)

OPTION 12

14 Stacy's Soy Crisps (**Green**)

Grapes (**Free Fuel**)

OPTION 13

1 medium apple (**Free Fuel**)

1 tablespoon peanut butter (**Green**)

OPTION 14

4 ounces fruit-flavored, fat-free yogurt (**Green**)

1 cup strawberries (**Free Fuel**)

Red Light, Green Light, Eat Right

Garlic and Sun-Dried Tomato Hummus and Pitas

Chickpeas are loaded with fiber. This recipe spices up hummus with garlic and sun-dried tomato for a flavorful dip.

MAKES 3 SERVINGS ■ EACH SERVING (¼ CUP HUMMUS + 4 WHOLE WHEAT PITA WEDGES) = 1 YELLOW

PREP TIME: 5–7 minutes
COOK TIME: 6 minutes
READY TIME: 11–13 minutes

Vegetable cooking spray

2 (6-inch) whole wheat pitas

¼ cup water

2 tablespoons chopped oil-packed sun-dried tomato halves

½ teaspoon salt

¼ teaspoon freshly ground black pepper

2 garlic cloves

1 (15-ounce) can chickpeas, drained

1. Preheat the oven to 425°F.

2. Coat a baking sheet with cooking spray. Cut each pita into 6 even-size wedges and place on the baking sheet. Bake for 6 minutes or until golden.

3. Combine the water, tomatoes, salt, pepper, garlic, and chickpeas in a food processor and process until smooth.

4. Place the hummus in a bowl and serve with the pita wedges.

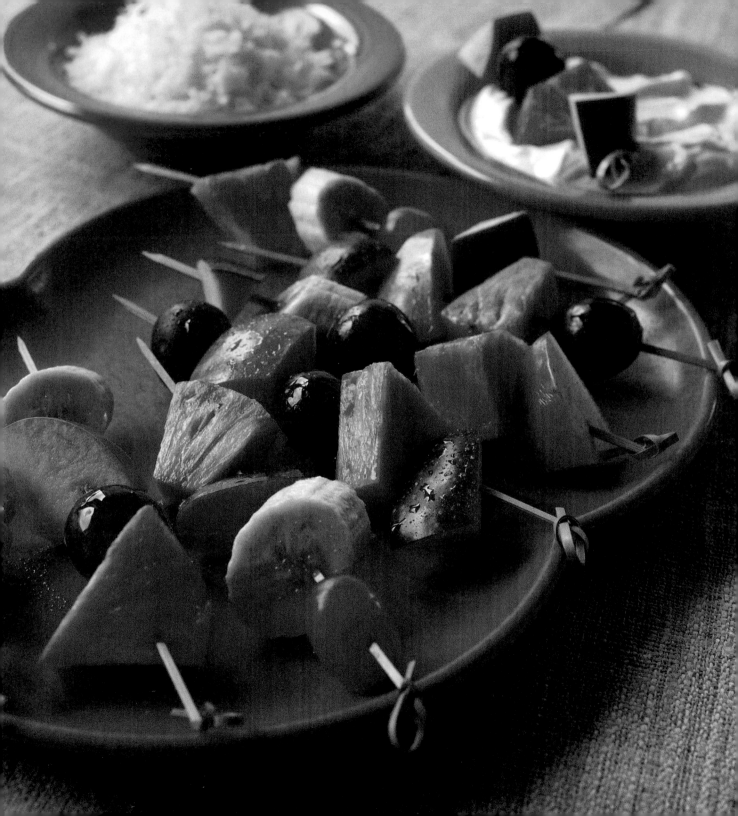

Fun Fruit Kebobs

Here's a recipe that turns snacktime into playtime. Kids get to spear pieces of fruit, then roll them in yogurt and coconut for a yummy snack.

MAKES APPROXIMATELY 6 SKEWERS ■ EACH SERVING (2 SKEWERS) = 1 GREEN

PREP TIME: 10 minutes
COOK TIME: None
READY TIME: 10 minutes

⅓ cup red seedless grapes

⅓ cup green seedless grapes

1 apple

1 banana

⅔ cup pineapple chunks

2 wooden skewer sticks

1 cup fat-free yogurt

¼ cup shredded dried coconut

1. Prepare the fruit by washing the grapes, washing and cutting the apple into small squares, peeling the banana and cutting it into chunks, and cutting the pineapple into chunks (if it's fresh).

2. Place all the pieces on a large plate.

3. Spread the shredded coconut on another large plate.

4. Slide pieces of fruit onto two wooden skewers to design your own kebobs. Put as much fruit as you want on each skewer.

5. Hold the kebob at both ends and roll it in the yogurt, then roll it in the coconut.

Frozen Yogurt Pops

Children love frozen pops. Here's a fast way to make your own ice pops using fruit-flavored yogurt. After freezing, they're ready anytime—for snacks or dessert. They're an easy way to help your children get one of their three daily servings of dairy.

MAKES 1 POP ■ EACH SERVING (1 POP) = 1 GREEN

PREP TIME: 5 minutes
COOK TIME: None
READY TIME: Next day

4 ounces low-fat fruit-flavored
    yogurt
Chopped fruit
Popsicle sticks

1. In a bowl, mix together the yogurt and fruit.

2. Fill a small paper cup with the yogurt-fruit mixture and cover with aluminum foil.

3. Insert a Popsicle stick through the foil in the middle of the cup and freeze overnight.

4. Slide the pops out of the paper cups and enjoy.

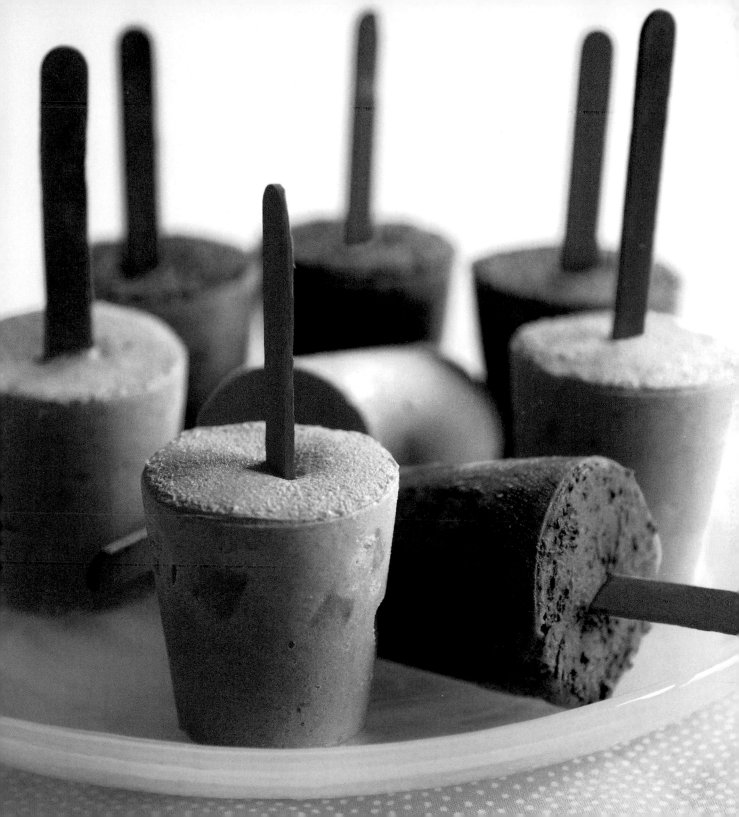

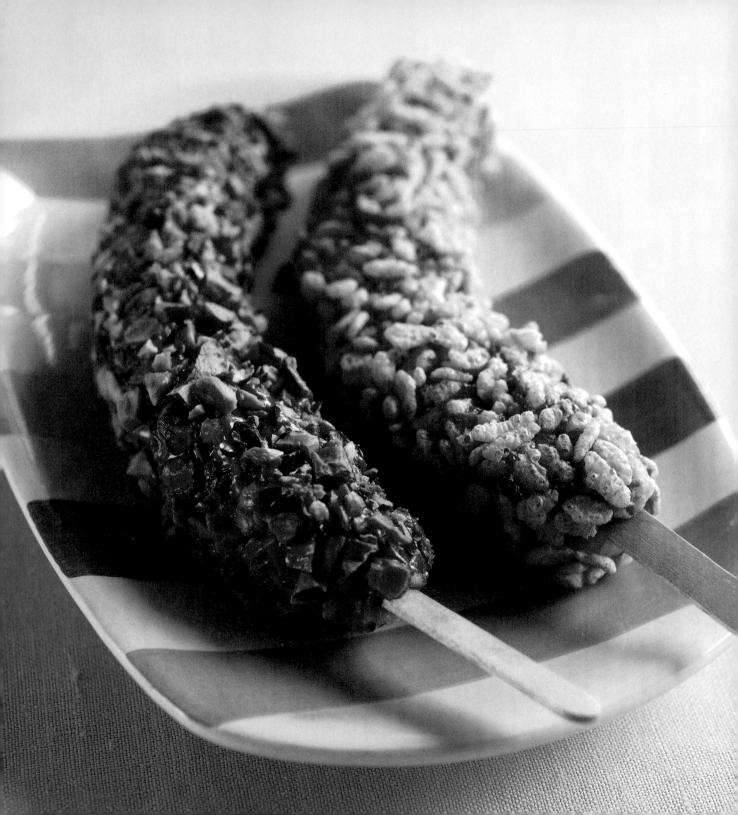

Banana Krispie/Nut Pops

Bananas are such a terrific Free Fuel—full of potassium and other minerals, plus energy-boosting carbs. There are so many dishes you can make with them, including this yummy frozen pop that is as much fun to make as it is to eat.

MAKES 2 POPS ■ EACH SERVING WITH RICE KRISPIES = 1 GREEN ; WITH ALMONDS = 1 YELLOW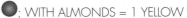

PREP TIME: 5 minutes
COOK TIME: None
READY TIME: Next day

1 banana

Popsicle sticks

1 tablespoon peanut butter

½ cup Rice Krispies or
   3 tablespoons crushed
   almonds

1. Peel a banana and cut off the tip at one end. Insert a Popsicle stick into the cut end.

2. Spread the peanut butter on the banana.

3. Roll the "pop" in Rice Krispies or almonds.

4. Wrap each pop in waxed paper and freeze overnight.

5. Cut banana in half width-wise and serve.

Bugs on a Log

There's nothing more fun to children than edible art. And with this recipe, they create the art and then get to eat it. What a great way to help your kids get the nutrition they need!

MAKES 3 SERVINGS ■ EACH SERVING (1 LOG) = 1 GREEN

PREP TIME: 5 minutes
COOK TIME: None
READY TIME: 5 minutes

6 celery sticks (3 stalks, washed and chopped in half)

1 tablespoon peanut butter

Raisins

1. Spread the celery sticks with the peanut butter.

2. Top each log with 6 raisins.

VARIATION: If your child has nut allergies, try substituting 3 tablespoons hummus for the peanut butter and black olives for the raisins (1 serving is still a **Green Light**). This makes a great snack for parents and older kids, too!

DETOUR

During the week, children eat 18 percent of their total daily calories while watching TV; on weekends, 26 percent of their daily calories are consumed in front of the television.[1] Interestingly, a person's metabolic rate is lower while watching television than while staring at a blank wall. Researchers aren't sure why, but they speculate that flashing lights may put you into a hypnotic-like state or that you are so engrossed in the show that you fidget less. Either way, watching television is the worst thing a child can do in terms of calorie burn. Excessive TV watching turns kids into Screen Beans!

DON'T BE A SCREEN BEAN!

Not only are Screen Beans inactive and metabolically ineffi-cient, they are exposed to an average of 40,000 commercials a year, mostly for high-calorie and high-fat foods. Why do companies spend so much money on child-targeted advertising campaigns? They work! Commercials prompt kids to crave these unhealthy foods.[2] The lesson here: Monitor how much TV your kids watch—and watch their weight go down! And *never* let your kids mindlessly snack in front of the TV.

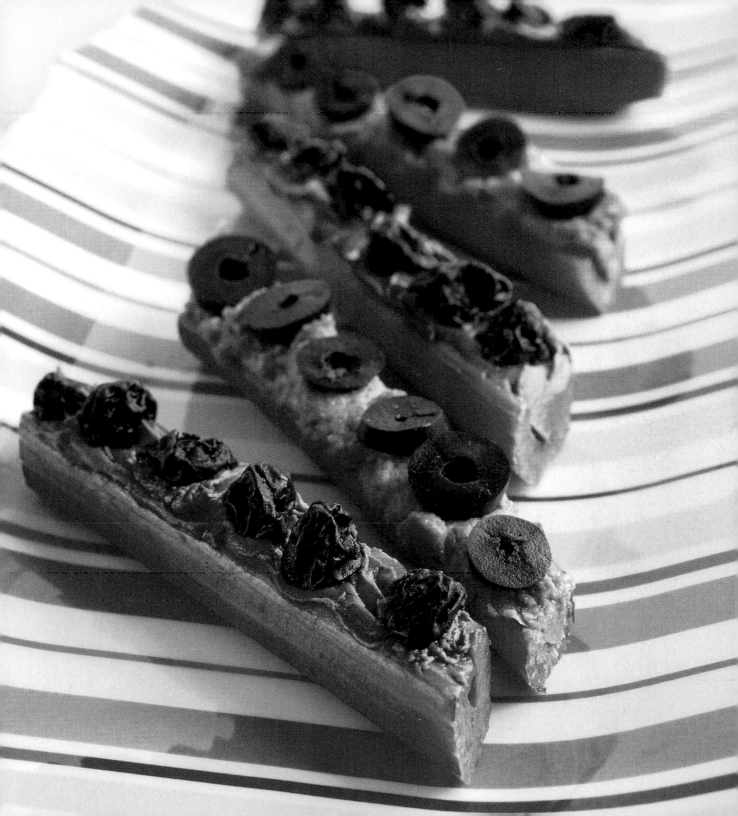

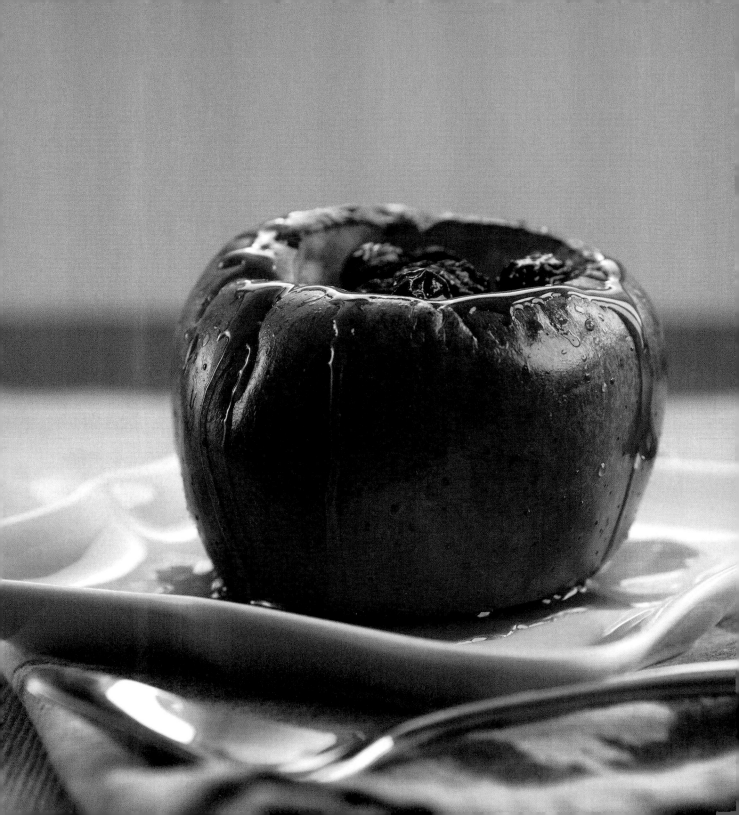

Baked Apple

Apples are a terrific source of fiber. Here's a way to turn a regular apple into a sweet treat.

MAKES 1 BAKED APPLE ■ EACH SERVING (1 APPLE) = *FREE FUEL*

PREP TIME: 10 minutes
COOK TIME: 30 minutes
READY TIME: 40 minutes

1 medium apple

Vegetable cooking spray

½ teaspoon Splenda brown sugar

6 raisins

1. Preheat the oven to 400°F.

2. Remove the apple core and place the apple in a small baking dish that has been sprayed with cooking spray.

3. Mix the Splenda, brown sugar, and raisins and place mixture in the center of the apple.

4. Place the small baking dish in a larger oven-safe dish that has been filled one-quarter full with boiling water. Bake until soft, about 30 minutes.

5. Several times during baking, spoon the liquid over the apple.

From the time you become a parent until you pack your kids off for college, snack foods will make up a sizable portion of what your child eats, so get them in the habit early of choosing wholesome snacks. Healthy snack habits are a great way to motivate kids to make nutritious choices throughout their lifetimes.

TRAFFIC TIP

Create a "Healthy Shelf"

Jimmy, a former patient of mine, was a good-looking kid who loved baseball, but his sports involvement was pretty much restricted to sitting on the sidelines. In school, no one wanted him on their team because his extra pounds made him slow and awkward. His classmates would tease him on the playground when he tried to run. After-school snacking was a problem for Jimmy, age 12. His parents both worked, so he was home alone after school. Jimmy used to rummage in the kitchen, eating whatever he could find. His mom kept chips and cookies in the house "because Dad liked them."

So the first step for this family was clearing out the junk food—if it's there, kids will find it. Next, I advised Jimmy's mom to make a "healthy shelf" in the cupboard and a "healthy drawer" in the fridge. She put all the Green Light snacks in these areas. The healthy shelf contained 100-calorie packs, pretzels, and air-popped popcorn. The healthy drawer contained cheese sticks, fat-free cheese, yogurt, fruits, and veggies. Now Jimmy rummages around all he wants as long as he selects from the healthy shelf and the healthy drawer. He loves having choices, and his mom loves that he snacks on healthy foods.

Try this in your own home. Create an accessible healthy shelf and healthy drawer in your kitchen and in your refrigerator. Your kids will grab what is quickest, but with the preparation already done, they will also be grabbing the healthy snacks. There is really no need to have chips and candy in the house; these foods should be special treats. Another benefit of the healthy shelf is that you don't have to get up every time your child is hungry (which in my house is all the time!). As for Jimmy, he lost those extra pounds and now plays third base in a baseball league.

7

● ● ●

DINNER DESTINATIONS

One of the best ways to help your child lose weight, maintain normal weight, and stay healthy is to schedule regular family mealtimes. Sure, I know how hard it can be to avoid eating dinner in "shifts" (I often work late), with kids eating earlier in the evening than parents, or to fit in a quick meal between sports and activity schedules. But as hectic as our lives may be, it's worthwhile to sit down and share dinner as a family. In fact, a Harvard Medical School study of more than 16,000 children between the ages of 9 and 14 found that kids who regularly ate dinner with their families generally had more healthful eating patterns than those who ate by themselves. Not only were they more likely to eat at least five daily servings of fruits and/or vegetables, but their intake of fried foods and soda was lower and their consumption of fiber, calcium, fat, and essential vitamins (such as C, E, and B vitamins) was higher.

Other research has suggested that family dinners lower the risk of eating disorders and obesity among children and teens. Kids who sit down to frequent family dinners are less likely to try drugs, drink alcohol, or smoke, and they're more likely to get better grades, according to the National Center on Addiction and Substance Abuse at Columbia University.

Too often children are free to feed themselves at

dinnertime because Mom and Dad aren't yet home. I worked with a family last year, the McKays, whose teenaged kids—Allen, 15, and Rebecca, 16—were grabbing dinner from fast-food restaurants or ordering pizza at home because Mom and Dad worked late and the kids were hungry by 6:00. Even when Mrs. McKay prepared healthy dinners and left them in the fridge for the kids to reheat, Allen and Rebecca didn't always eat them, or they'd eat their mom's cooking *and* a bunch of junk food because no one was monitoring them. Both Allen and Rebecca had been steadily gaining weight and were at least 20 pounds overweight when the family came to see me for help. The McKays didn't know what to do, yet they knew if they didn't do something, their children might face a lifetime of social challenges, low self-esteem, and a significantly higher risk of developing major health problems.

I suggested that the family move their mealtime to a later hour so that everyone could eat together. Because Mom and Dad were home by 7:00, the family agreed that dinner would be at 7:30. So that Allen and Rebecca wouldn't be too hungry by dinnertime, we took a **Green Light** from their dinner allotment and moved it to their afternoon snack, which gave them extra fuel to tide them over until dinner. The whole family loved the new schedule, and dinnertime became an opportunity to talk about the day and enjoy a meal together. And Mom and Dad could keep an eye on what Allen and Rebecca were eating. The whole family began cooking and eating healthier dinners—and losing weight.

As the McKays discovered, eating dinner together sets the stage for positive family bonding experiences. It's a chance to catch up on what's going on in everyone's lives. In my family, we play a game during dinner. We go around the table, and each of us answers the question: What was the best part of your day today? It's a great way to get the whole family talking—and enjoying a healthy meal together. Children then know they get to share a portion of their day with the family, and parents get to learn more about what's going on with their kids.

The Healthiest-Ever Dinners

Because kids are usually very hungry at dinner, it's a perfect time to serve healthy foods like salads and vegetables. Ideally, a child's dinner should include high-quality foods: a lean protein; unprocessed carbohydrates such as potatoes, sweet potatoes, or whole grains; and plenty of vegetables (**Free Fuel**). There are lots of options available for lean meats and healthy, nutritious carbs.

HEALTHY DINNER MAKEOVERS

MEATS		
●	●	●
4 oz ground beef (75% lean), cooked	3 oz ground beef (90% lean), cooked	2 oz ground beef (95% lean), cooked
2½ oz regular steak	3 oz skirt steak or 3 oz lean steak	2 oz veal loin
1½ slices brisket	3 oz flank steak	4 slices roast beef lunch meat
1 link chorizo sausage	1½ links Italian sausage	1 link vegetable sausage
1 large meatball	3 medium-size turkey meatballs	3 veggie meatballs
4-oz hamburger patty, restaurant	3-oz hamburger patty, made with 90% lean beef	2-oz hamburger patty, made with 93% lean beef
STARCHY CARBOHYDRATES		
●	●	●
16 french fries, fried	10 Tater Tots	10 french fries, frozen, baked without fat
1 cup corn pudding	1 cup cream-style corn	¾ cup corn kernels
2 potato skins	½ cup garlic mashed potatoes	2 small new potatoes, boiled
Baked potato with cheese sauce	⅔ cup potatoes au gratin	4 oz of a baked potato
1 slice sweet potato pie	½ cup candied sweet potato	4 oz of a baked sweet potato
1 cup fried rice	1 cup white rice	½ cup brown rice

The above chart shows just how simple it is to turn an unhealthy dinner into a Green Light dinner, and the Appendix at the back of the book lists hundreds more choices for healthy dinners. Take a peek at your options and get creative!

Inviting Kids into the Kitchen

I've been working with a family, the Millers, whose two children, Patrick, 8, and Kathy, 6, have experienced great success on their game plans. One reason is because Mom and Dad welcome little helpers in the kitchen. Yes, it can be a bit more work to get meals on

Dinner Planning

Is it late afternoon and you still have no idea what to make for dinner? Like any meal, dinner can be stressful when you don't plan ahead. Here are some simple tips to make dinner planning easier.

- Whenever possible, shop in bulk. Make a shopping trip to a warehouse store like BJ's or Costco for essential pantry foods that are nonperishable as well as items that can be kept frozen. Such foods would include chicken breasts, extralean ground meat, fish, frozen vegetables, frozen fruit, canned beans, canned sauce, brown rice, whole wheat pasta, potatoes, and whole wheat bread or rolls.

- Buy prepared produce when in a rush; this saves you time and encourages you to eat your recommended servings each day. Look for prewashed, precut salads, carrots, peppers, or other veggies of choice. Prepared vegetables may cost a little bit more than whole vegetables, but it's still cheaper—and healthier—than take-out.

- Divide meats into serving sizes before freezing so you can easily defrost one dinner's worth a few hours before a meal.

- Prepare meals in advance. If you have time on a Sunday afternoon, prepare two meals for the week and keep them refrigerated until needed.

- Make big batches of menu items you know you will repeat during the week. This way, you avoid cooking twice. For example, if Monday and Wednesday dinners include rice, make enough for the 2 days.

- Use a slow cooker; it's especially handy in the fall and winter for meals such as stews, soups, and hearty meat dishes.

- Broil or grill fish for a quick, low-calorie meal. Top with fresh lemon, black pepper, or even fruit salsa.

- Out of groceries? Try breakfast for dinner. Eggs are a convenient and inexpensive form of protein. Make an omelet with fat-free cheese and any vegetables you have on hand, then supplement with a slice of whole wheat toast.

- Hot sandwiches for dinner are also a healthy choice. If you have a panini maker or sandwich press, you can create a fun, healthy dinner using lean proteins and whole grain bread.

- Skinless precut meats and poultry are great for making quick meals. Try using them to make kebobs, stews, and stir-fried dishes with veggies.

Get Growing!

For many kids, the concept of "vegetables" means little more than a plate of french fries or a bag of corn chips. The truth is, our kids tend to see vegetables only after they've been processed and made into something else. One excellent way to teach youngsters about vegetables is to plant a garden in your backyard. Your kids can plant the seeds, tend the seedlings, and harvest veggies for dinner. Kids love to play in the dirt anyway, and they're more likely to eat what they've grown themselves. So give your kids some beans or tomatoes to plant and watch what happens at the dinner table.

If you're short on space, consider planting a small container garden. Or simply grow some veggies or herbs in a pot on your kitchen windowsill. Additionally, you can sprout almost any bean or seed, although alfalfa is one of the most familiar. Sprouts grow fast, provide crunchy nutrition, and require minimal effort. The idea is to teach your kids that veggies come from soil—not a drive-thru!

the table when the kids are involved in preparing food, but the short-term inconvenience is worth the long-term benefits. The Millers knew their children needed to lose weight and wanted them to learn about healthy nutrition. By taking Patrick and Kathy along on grocery shopping trips, allowing them to help select recipes, and letting them get their hands dirty in the kitchen, the Millers found that their children have enthusiastically embraced their new meal plans.

The Miller kids are young, but Mom lets them do as much as they can. She gives them small jobs such as washing veggies, spinning salad, or stirring ingredients in a bowl so they feel involved and important. Mom takes care of anything that involves handling a knife or being near the stove. As a result, when the meal is placed on the table, everyone feels a sense of pride, and the kids are even willing to try new foods. During dinner, they each take turns talking about their day. In fact, dinnertime has become one of the Miller family's favorite parts of the day.

Expose Your Children to New Foods

What if your child turns up his nose at brussels sprouts or couscous the first, second, or even third time you serve it? Keep trying. We know from research that it often takes as many as 10 to 15 trials before children develop a liking for a new food. Continue to encourage your child to try new foods, different tastes, and unfamiliar textures; don't allow your child to make the decisions about what he will or won't eat.

Healthy eating habits must be taught at a young age. Children who are exposed to a variety of foods during childhood are more likely to learn to enjoy those foods as adults, even if they didn't like them as kids. Eating different foods ensures that your children are getting all the nutrients they need to grow.

Tips for Introducing New Foods

When parents share their frustration with me about the limited taste buds of their picky eaters, I encourage them to keep introducing new foods to their family's diet using the following pointers:

- **Lead by example.** Try new foods yourself. When your kids see you enjoying healthy foods, they're more likely to want to try them, too. Make it a point to let your kids know when you try something new and find that it's delicious. They'll want a taste!
- **Be positive.** I present foods to my children with enthusiasm. Instead of saying, "You must eat your green beans," I say, "Wow! We have green beans today. Yummy!" Whenever possible, come up with fun games and positive associations about the food on their plates. For example, in my family, we call broccoli "trees." I used to tell my son, "I can't believe you're eating a tree!" He would giggle. Best of all, he loves broccoli.
- **Don't force-feed.** The fastest way to foster dislike of a particular food is to force your kids to eat it or punish them for not eating it. You don't want the dinner table to be a battleground. Food should be a source of nourishment, bonding, and enjoyment—not tears.
- **Institute the "two-bite rule."** Tell your children they must try two bites of each new food they are served. If they don't like the food, they do not have to eat the rest. However, they do need to eat two bites each time it is served. Chances are that, over time, your children will learn to like it. Once you've introduced a new food, try to wait at least 1 week before serving it again. My kids have grown up with this rule.
- **Be flexible.** No child is going to be excited to try every single new food, and in general the two-bite rule should always apply. But there are limits. My son (who is a healthy eater) absolutely hates salmon. So when the rest of us eat salmon, I make

Have Your Kids Tried These Yummy Whole Grains?

Get your family in the habit of enjoying a full range of whole grains. A whole grain typically has all three parts of the grain seed, or kernel. Studies show that eating at least three whole grain servings daily can reduce the risk of heart disease, help with weight control, and prevent many chronic diseases. Try introducing the following foods into your children's diet. These grains can be included in soups or served as side dishes, and many of them are delicious as breakfast food.

Barley	Couscous	Triticale
Brown rice	Millet	Whole wheat bread
Buckwheat	Oats	Wild rice
Bulgur	Quinoa	
Corn kernels (popcorn)	Sprouted grains	

him a peanut butter and jelly sandwich. He is excused from the two-bite rule for this particular food that he truly can't stomach. The idea is to be firm but reasonable. When he tries to get out of the rule for chicken (which isn't his favorite, but he doesn't hate it), the answer is 100 percent no.

As a parent, it's up to you to decide what foods will be kept in the house and prepared for meals, as well as when those meals will be served. If possible, try to serve dinner at the same time every day to encourage healthy habits. Once your family gathers for a meal, eliminate distractions. Turn off the television and computer. And no phone calls or texting at the dinner table! In addition to focusing on the food and conversation, you will be teaching your children how to behave properly at mealtime.

What If Your Child Is a Picky Eater?

Picky eaters usually fall into one of two camps: They either eat small portions of foods at a time or eat the

Dinner in a Hurry

Here is a list of my 10 favorite quick-fix dinners.

- Ready-to-eat rotisserie chicken from the grocery store (Just pull off the skin.)
- 2 eggs or egg whites on reduced-calorie whole grain toast
- Chicken quesadilla made with whole wheat tortillas, fat-free shredded cheese, and grilled chicken strips
- Whole wheat pasta with turkey meatballs and marinara sauce
- Frozen thin-crust pizza crust topped with marinara sauce and fat-free cheese
- 97 percent fat-free hot dogs, boiled, served with baked frozen french fries
- Peanut butter sandwich on reduced-calorie whole wheat bread
- Low-sodium canned soup, a whole grain roll, and a piece of fruit
- 1 slice of pizza and a fresh side salad
- Frozen Lean Cuisine entrée and a fresh side salad

same foods over and over and refuse to try anything new. Both of these behaviors are perfectly normal, so there is no need to worry if your child exhibits either tendency. New research is shedding light on how children's food preferences are formed and what parents can do to promote healthy eating. We know, for example, that kids have five times more taste buds than adults do, making them much more sensitive to the four main flavor sensations—sweet, sour, bitter, and salty. Here are my suggestions for dealing with picky eaters.

- **Take your kids' tastes into account.** Children generally gravitate mostly to sweet and salty tastes—which is one reason many kids shun vegetables. Try sprinkling a little grated fat-free cheese on vegetables. The salt in the cheese counteracts some of the bitterness. Or serve snacks of sweeter veggies, like baby carrots, red bell peppers, and grape tomatoes.

- **Don't be a short-order cook!** Fixing separate meals for every member of the family only reinforces a picky eater's habits. Each meal should contain some foods the kids like and some foods the adults like.

- **Don't bribe kids.** I don't believe in practices like promising ice cream as a reward for eating spinach. This only fuels the suspicion that there's something wrong with the spinach.

- **Have your picky eater sit with you,** or with a sibling who has developed a more adventurous palate, and introduce new smells and tastes as you share a meal. Teach your fussy child a new saying: "Eat a food you hate and you just might wind up with a food you love!"

- **Deal positively with refusals.** When all is said and done, some picky eaters will stubbornly refuse to eat the meal. Don't argue, yell, threaten, bribe, or otherwise get angry. Don't worry about your child missing a meal or two, either. Trust me: That child will get hungry later—so wrap up that meal and save it for when he or she is ready. Stay firm. Just don't give in and let kids eat junk instead!

Sitting Down to Dinner

Begin dinners with a salad with fat-free dressing or with a broth-based soup. Salads and soups are filling, so there's little chance that your kids will overeat or have too many second helpings. Get rid of huge dinner plates, too. Eating on small dishes—which look full even with small portions—tricks your brain into thinking you're eating a larger meal.

Take your time as you eat. It takes about 20 minutes for your body to realize it's full. Meals should last at least that long. If your children finish eating too quickly and are still hungry, make them wait before you serve seconds. Distract them with conversation or offer them more fruit and vegetables. But make sure it's been a full 20 minutes before they get seconds. Chances are they won't still be hungry 20 minutes after their initial request. If they are, they can have a small second portion—but make sure it is counted toward their traffic light allotment for the day.

As you plan dinner, always include **Free Fuel** in the form of a vegetable, either served raw or cooked without added fats. When it comes to the more caloric parts of the meal, such as the rice, pasta, or meat, make sure that what you put on your child's plate is equal to about one serving per person. If the recipe requires you to make more, or if you want to make extra for lunch the next day, pack away the leftovers *before* serving dinner. Then, if your children are still hungry, only the healthy options, such as the vegetables, remain on the table. Unwrapping and microwaving leftovers will seem like too much work. Choose foods based on your child's personalized eating plan.

What's for Dinner?

Here are some sample meal ideas for healthy, balanced dinners. Remember, you can always do some of the prep work in advance the night before so that you reduce your time spent in the kitchen on weeknights and get dinner onto the table more quickly.

SAMPLE DINNERS

OPTION 1

1 DELICIOUS BEEF BURGER (page 124) (**Yellow**)

1 light whole wheat hamburger bun (**Green**)

½ cup green peas (**Free Fuel**)

Small tossed salad with 3 tablespoons fat-free Italian dressing (**Free Fuel**)

OPTION 2

BAKED FISH STICKS (page 127) (**Green, Green, Green**)

1 cup stir-fried vegetables, prepared with vegetable cooking spray (**Free Fuel**)

1 serving POTATO WEDGES (page 128) (**Green**)

OPTION 3

1 cup whole wheat spaghetti with marinara sauce (**Green, Green**)

⅓ cup ground chicken meatballs (**Green**)

1 cup broccoli (**Free Fuel**)

OPTION 4

1 CHICKEN FAJITA (page 131) (**Green, Green, Green**)

½ cup black beans (**Green**)

Small tossed salad with 3 tablespoons fat-free Italian dressing (**Free Fuel**)

OPTION 5

2 ounces filet mignon (trimmed of fat) or other lean steak (**Yellow**)

⅔ cup homemade mashed potatoes, made with fat-free milk but without butter (**Green**)

Steamed veggies (**Free Fuel**)

OPTION 6

TILAPIA WITH LEMON, GARLIC, AND CAPERS (page 132) (**Green**)

Steamed green beans (**Free Fuel**)

½ cup whole wheat couscous (**Green**)

1 small tossed salad with 3 tablespoons fat-free Italian dressing (**Free Fuel**)

OPTION 7

HEALTHY PASTA AND VEGETABLE DISH (page 136) (**Green, Green, Green**)

OPTION 8

6 CHICKEN NUGGETS (page 135) (**Yellow**)

Steamed vegetables (**Free Fuel**)

2 FROSTY STRAWBERRY YOGURT CUPCAKES (page 144) (**Green**)

OPTION 9

Chinese takeout: ⅔ cup vegetables with pork (**Yellow**)

½ cup brown rice (**Green**)

OPTION 10

SHRIMP AND PASTA DINNER (page 137) (**Green, Green, Green**)

Small tossed salad with 3 tablespoons fat-free Italian dressing (**Free Fuel**)

OPTION 11

TACO DINNER (page 138) (**Green, Green, Green**)

OPTION 12

DR. DOLGOFF'S CHICKEN "PARM" (page 141) (**Green, Green, Green**)

Small tossed salad with 3 tablespoons fat-free Italian dressing (**Free Fuel**)

OPTION 13

CAESAR SALAD WITH CHICKEN (page 142) (**Green, Green, Green**)

OPTION 14

½ cup extra-lean beef stir-fry meat (**Green**)

⅔ cup stir-fried vegetables (**Green**)

1 serving APPLE CRISP (page 147) (**Green**)

Dinner Recipes

Like all family meals, dinner requires a bit of creativity, effort, and negotiation. But the results will be more than worthwhile when you look at your vibrant children and know they are fit, happy, and well adjusted—and that you had a hand in it through the food you put on the dinner table.

Delicious Beef Burger

Try making burgers using extra-lean meats spiced up with ingredients like fresh garlic, onions, and other herbs and spices. They are just as delicious as the full-fat version and much healthier for your family.

MAKES 4 SERVINGS ■ EACH SERVING (1 4-OUNCE BURGER) = 1 YELLOW
1 LIGHT WHOLE WHEAT BUN = 1 GREEN

PREP TIME: 5 minutes
COOK TIME: 10 minutes
READY TIME: 15 minutes

1 pound extra-lean ground beef
(95 percent lean)

¼ cup minced onion

½–1 garlic clove (as desired),
crushed

2 tablespoons minced fresh
parsley

2 tablespoons tomato sauce

1 tablespoon Worcestershire
sauce

1 egg white

1. In a large bowl, combine all the ingredients with a fork.

2. Form the mixture into four ¾-inch-thick patties.

3. Broil or grill for 5 to 6 minutes per side, to an internal temperature of 160°F.

4. Place a burger on a toasted bun and top with lettuce, tomato, and mustard or ketchup.

Red Light, Green Light, Eat Right

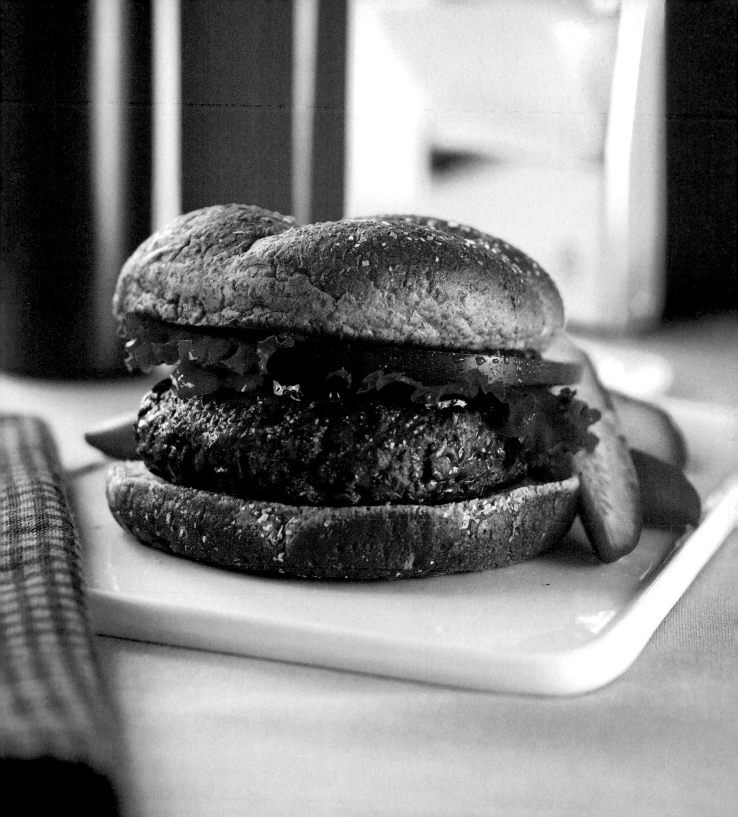

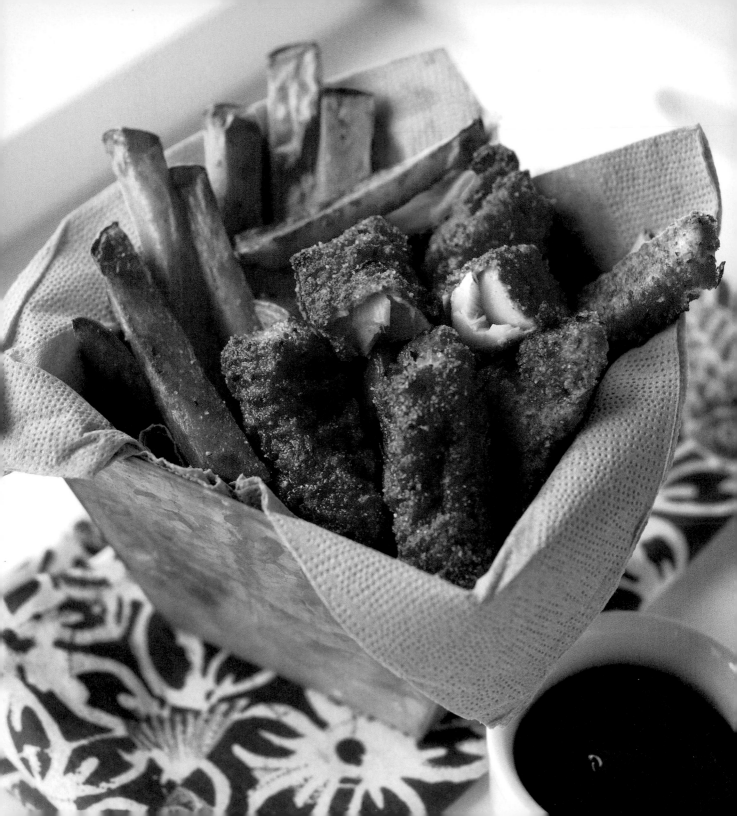

Baked Fish Sticks

Many of the kids I work with love fish sticks. But most frozen, store-bought varieties are loaded with fat and processed carbs. Here's a quick, easy way to make your own—minus all of the unhealthy additives.

MAKES 4 SERVINGS ■ EACH SERVING (4 OUNCES) = 3 GREENS

PREP TIME: 10 minutes
COOK TIME: 10 minutes
READY TIME: 20 minutes

Vegetable cooking spray
1 egg
3 egg whites
16 ounces halibut
¾ cup seasoned bread crumbs
4 tablespoons ketchup

1. Preheat the oven to 375°F.

2. Spray a baking sheet with cooking spray.

3. In a bowl, beat the egg and egg whites until mixed.

4. Slice the halibut into strips and dip the pieces into the egg mixture.

5. Place the fish in the bread crumbs and turn until coated.

6. Place the fish on the baking sheet and place in the oven.

7. Bake for about 10 minutes on each side or until the fish is opaque and flakes easily.

8. Serve with 1 tablespoon ketchup per serving.

Potato Wedges

This healthy version of the classic french fry is super delicious—and fat free. My family likes it when we prepare this dish with a mixture of regular potatoes and sweet potatoes.

MAKES 4 SERVINGS ■ EACH SERVING (4 OUNCES) = 1 GREEN

PREP TIME: 10 minutes

COOK TIME: 25 minutes

READY TIME: 35 minutes

4 potatoes (3½ ounces each)—combine white and sweet potatoes, if desired

2 egg whites, unbeaten

Vegetable cooking spray

Salt-free seasoning to taste

1. Preheat the oven to 425°F.

2. Cut the potatoes into wedges or, to make french fries, into thin slices.

3. Dip the wedges or slices into the unbeaten egg whites and place on a nonstick baking sheet coated with cooking spray.

4. Season with salt-free seasoning and bake for 25 minutes for wedges, 20 minutes for french fries, or until golden brown.

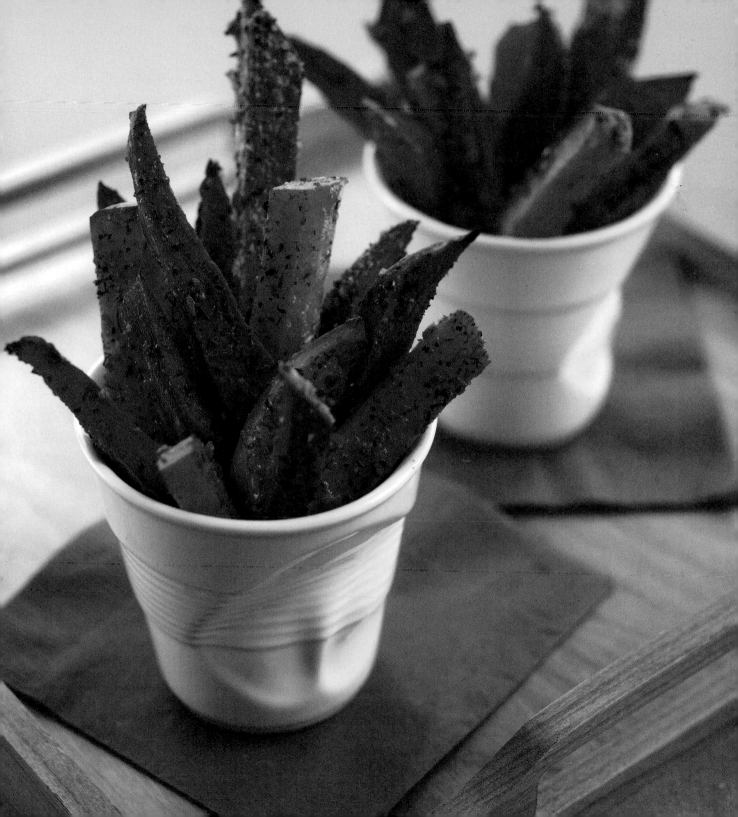

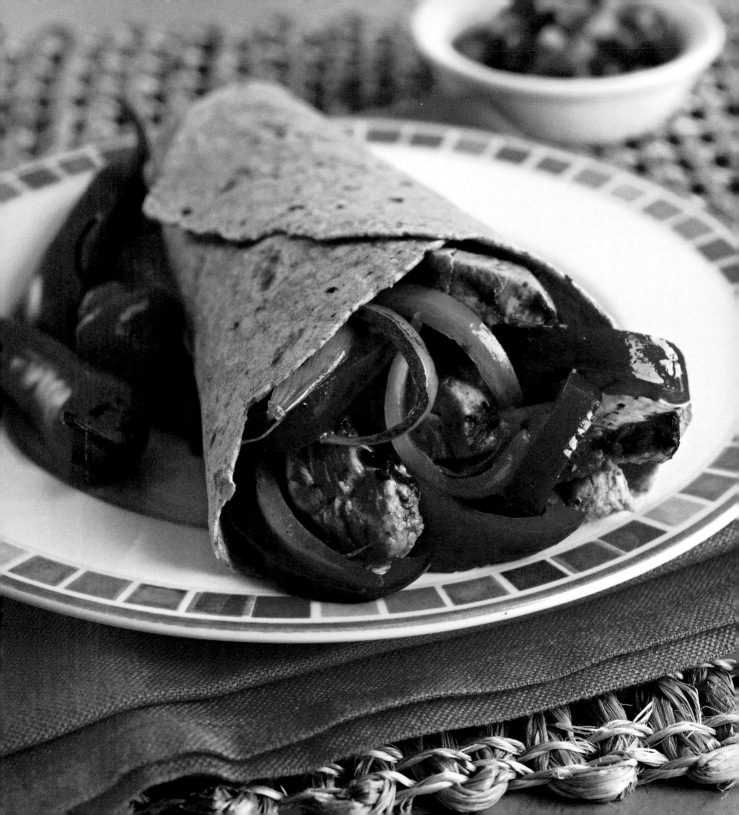

Chicken Fajitas

Here's a favorite Mexican dish—but one you can easily fix at home. Rather than cook your chicken in oil, use vegetable cooking spray. It works just as well yet contains much less fat.

MAKES 4 SERVINGS ■ EACH SERVING (1 FAJITA) = 3 GREENS

PREP TIME: 1 hour 10 minutes
COOK TIME: 5 minutes
READY TIME: 1 hour 15 minutes

16 ounces sliced grilled chicken

Packaged Mexican fajita
    seasoning

Vegetable cooking spray

1 small onion, sliced

2 small green bell peppers,
    sliced

4 (6-inch-diameter) whole
    wheat tortillas

1. Marinate the grilled chicken in the fajita seasoning according to package directions. Let marinate in the refrigerator for an hour.

2. Spray a skillet with cooking spray and sauté the onion and bell peppers until soft. Remove the veggies and set aside.

3. Spray the skillet with cooking spray again. Place a tortilla in the skillet, heating each side for about 3 seconds. Repeat with the other tortillas until all have been warmed.

4. Divide the chicken among the tortillas and top each with the pepper and onion mixture. Fold in the tortilla edges and serve.

Tilapia with Lemon, Garlic, and Capers

If you want your kids to eat more fish, try cooking a mild fish like tilapia. It will suit their developing palates, and it's a great source of protein.

MAKES 4 SERVINGS ■ EACH SERVING (1 SMALL FILLET) = 1 GREEN

PREP TIME: 5 minutes
COOK TIME: 12 minutes
READY TIME: 17 minutes

1 tablespoon olive oil

1 teaspoon minced garlic (about 2 cloves)

1–1½ pounds tilapia fillets or other thin white fish fillets (4 small fillets)

¼ teaspoon salt, or to taste

⅛ teaspoon ground black pepper, or to taste

Juice of ¾ lemon (about 2–3 tablespoons)

1 tablespoon capers, drained, or 1 tablespoon chopped green olives

1 teaspoon lemon zest

1. Warm the olive oil in a skillet. Add the garlic and cook for 30 seconds, until fragrant.

2. Add the fish fillets to the pan and season them with a little of the salt and pepper. Cook them for 3 to 4 minutes, depending on the thickness of the fillets, until the bottoms start to brown.

3. Flip the fillets, pour the lemon juice over them, and season the second side with salt and pepper.

4. Top the fish with the capers. Cook for another 3 to 4 minutes. When the fish is white throughout and flakes easily, remove it to a plate and serve.

5. Top the fish with fresh lemon zest and spoon lemon juice and caper mixture from the skillet over the top.

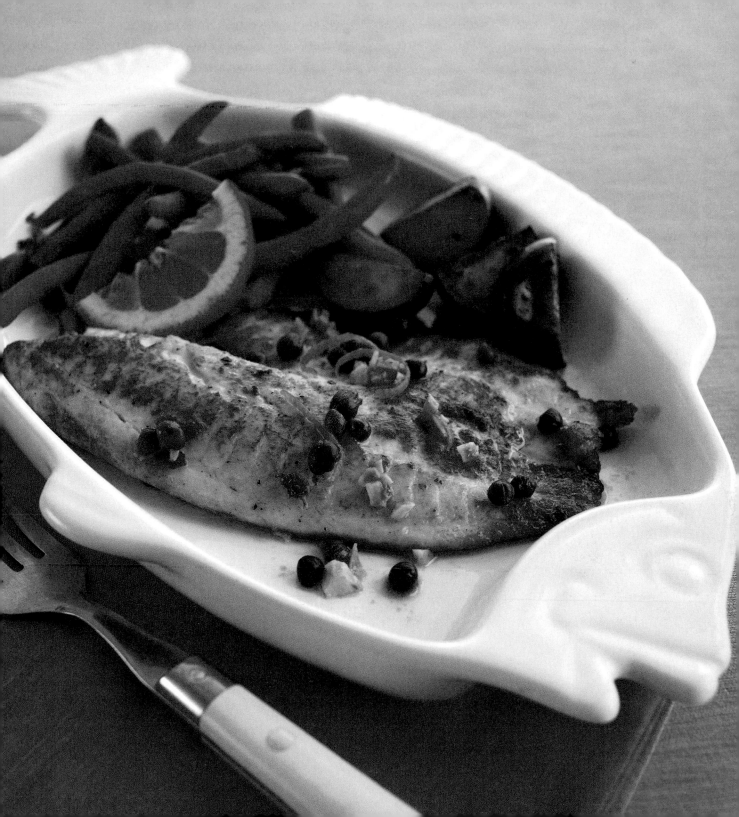

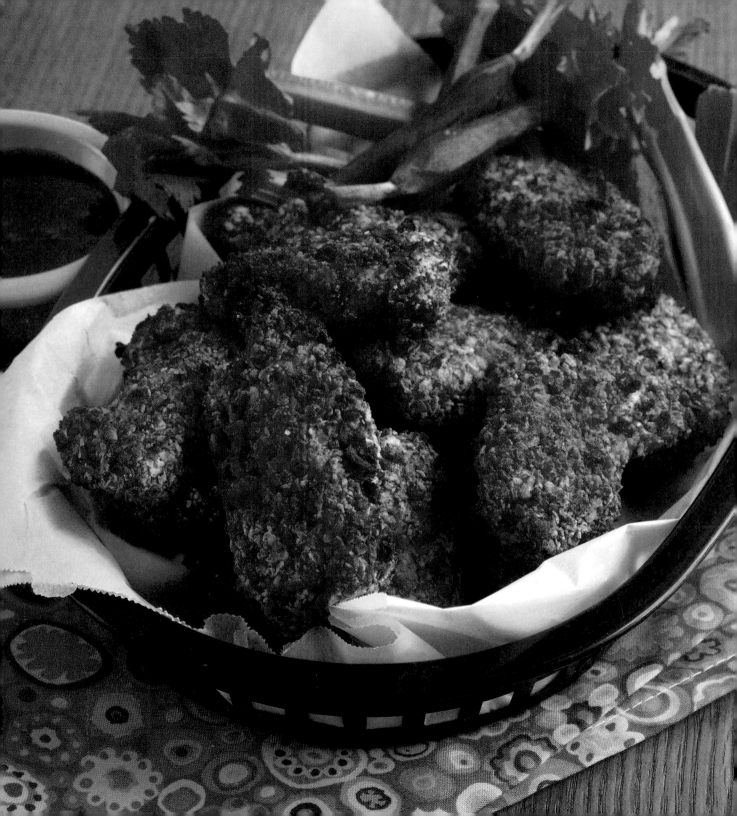

Chicken Nuggets

As a pediatrician and mother of two young children, I know how much kids love chicken nuggets! Yet most chicken nuggets are high in fat. This healthy version is crispy on the outside and tender on the inside, and tastes better than any chicken nuggets you can get from a drive-thru.

MAKES 5 SERVINGS ■ EACH SERVING (3 OUNCES) = 1 YELLOW

PREP TIME: 15 minutes
COOK TIME: 5 minutes
READY TIME: 20 minutes

Vegetable cooking spray

1 cup instant mashed potato flakes

1½ tablespoons grated Parmesan cheese

1½ teaspoons paprika

1½ teaspoons onion powder

½ teaspoon salt

Whites of 2 large eggs

1 pound boneless, skinless chicken breast halves, cut crosswise into 1-inch-wide strips

2 tablespoons honey (optional)

1 cup fat-free plain yogurt (optional)

1. Heat the oven to 500°F.

2. Set a wire rack on a baking sheet. Coat the rack with cooking spray.

3. Mix the potato flakes, cheese, paprika, onion powder, and salt on a piece of waxed paper.

4. In a medium bowl, beat the egg whites with a fork until slightly frothy.

5. Add the chicken to the egg whites and toss to coat.

6. Dredge the chicken strips in the potato mixture to cover.

7. Place the chicken strips on the prepared rack and lightly spray the top of the chicken with cooking spray.

8. Bake for 3 minutes, turn the strips over, spray again, and bake for another 1 to 3 minutes, until the chicken is crisp and cooked through.

9. Serve with honey or yogurt as dipping sauces, if desired.

Healthy Pasta and Vegetable Dish

I love this recipe because it delivers protein, high-fiber carbs, and plenty of **Free Fuel** veggies—all in one dish. It can be served hot or cold—save leftovers for tomorrow's lunch!

MAKES 4 SERVINGS ■

EACH SERVING (1⅓ CUPS PASTA + LOTS OF VEGETABLES + 2 OUNCES CHICKEN) = 3 GREENS

PREP TIME: 5 minutes

COOK TIME: 25 minutes

READY TIME: 30 minutes

3–4 chicken breasts, marinated in low-sodium herb seasoning

1 box whole wheat or brown rice pasta

3 cups frozen mixed vegetables

Vegetable cooking spray

Ground black pepper to taste

1 garlic clove, minced

½ cup fat-free Italian dressing

1. Remove the chicken breasts from the marinade and grill them on an indoor or outdoor grill until cooked through.

2. Cook the pasta according to the package directions.

3. Partially defrost the vegetables in the microwave, then sauté the veggies in a skillet lightly coated with cooking spray, adding black pepper and garlic to taste.

4. In a large bowl, combine the pasta and vegetables, then add the dressing and coat thoroughly.

5. Cut the chicken breasts into cubes and serve on top of the pasta.

Shrimp and Pasta Dinner

If your kids love pasta, here's a way to make it healthy and full of great taste—simply add shrimp and marinara sauce. Serve it with a salad and you've got a nutritious dinner for the whole family.

MAKES 4 SERVINGS ■ EACH SERVING (1 CUP + 6 SHRIMP) = 3 GREENS

PREP TIME: 5 minutes
COOK TIME: 20 minutes
READY TIME: 25 minutes

8 ounces uncooked whole wheat pasta

Vegetable cooking spray

24 large shrimp, cleaned and deveined

1 garlic clove, minced

2 cups marinara sauce

Salt and ground black pepper to taste

1. Prepare the pasta according to the package directions.

2. Spray a skillet with vegetable cooking spray, then sauté the shrimp and garlic until the shrimp is cooked through. Add salt and black pepper to taste.

3. In a large bowl, mix the pasta and shrimp together.

4. Heat the marinara sauce and spoon it over the pasta and shrimp mixture. Serve immediately.

Taco Dinner

Kids love assembling their own tacos. Give them healthy toppings to choose from and you'll sneak some extra veggies into their day!

MAKES 4 SERVINGS ■ EACH SERVING (2 TACOS) = 3 GREENS

PREP TIME: 2 minutes
COOK TIME: 15 minutes
READY TIME: 17 minutes

16 ounces extra-lean ground beef

2 tablespoons taco seasoning, prepared according to package directions

8 (6-inch) corn tortillas

1 cup fat-free shredded cheese

1 cup chopped lettuce

1 cup chopped tomato

1 cup salsa

1 cup chopped green bell pepper

1. Sauté the beef with the taco seasoning until cooked through.

2. Warm the tortillas in the microwave for approximately 30 seconds or until just softened.

3. Spoon beef into each of the warm tortillas.

4. Let the kids top their own tacos with the cheese, lettuce, tomato, salsa, and bell pepper.

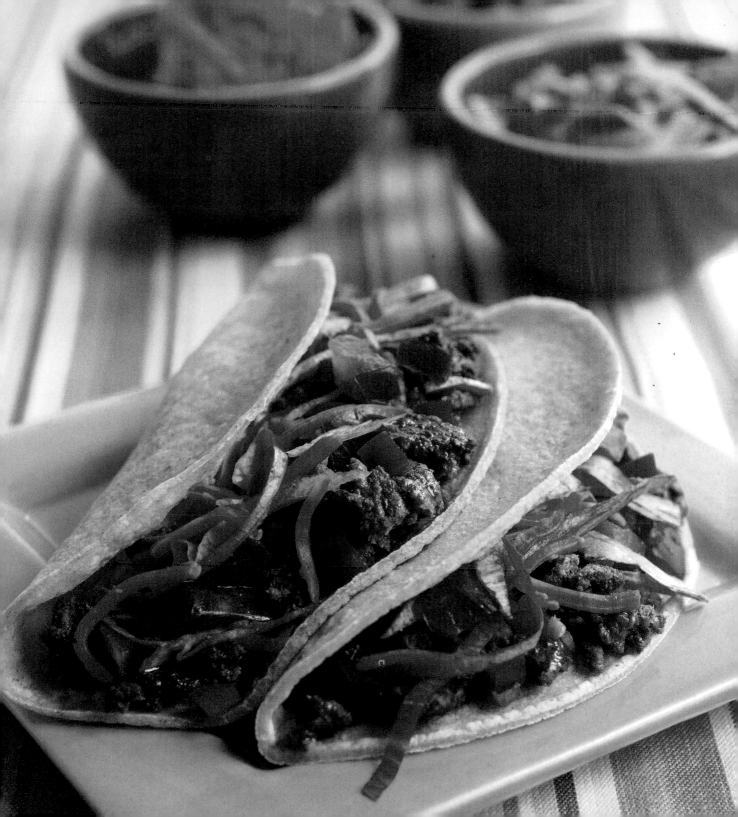

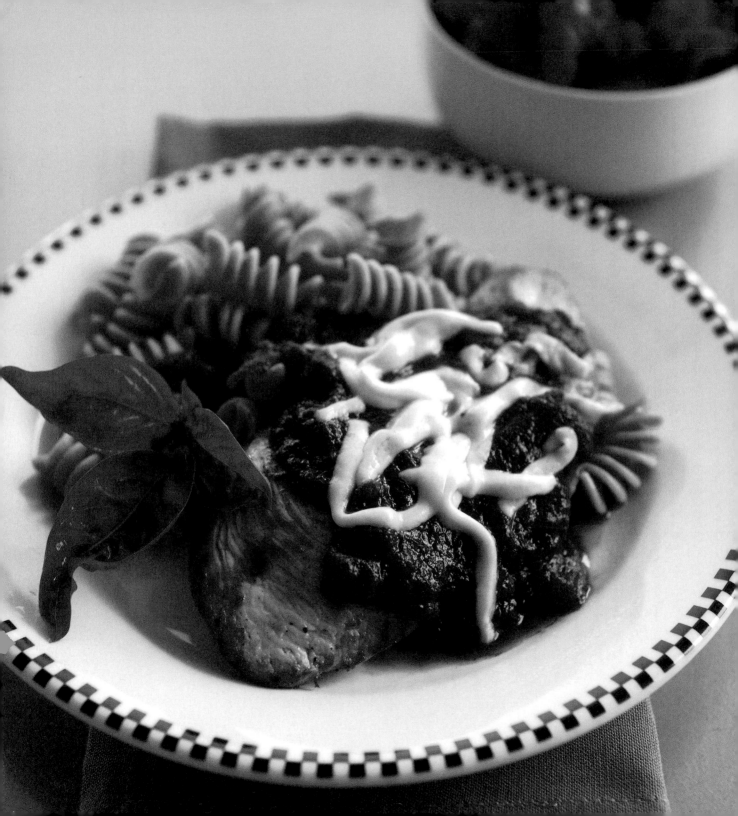

Dr. Dolgoff's Chicken "Parm"

We have this Green Light comfort food for dinner at my house frequently, and no one ever tires of it because it's so flavorful and satisfying.

MAKES 4 SERVINGS ■ EACH SERVING (3 OUNCES CHICKEN + ⅔ CUP PASTA) = 3 GREENS

PREP TIME: 5 minutes
COOK TIME: 30 minutes
READY TIME: 35 minutes

12 ounces chicken breast

1 cup marinara sauce

2 cups fat-free mozzarella

2⅔ cups whole wheat pasta,
    cooked according to package
    directions

1. Preheat the oven to 350°F. Place the chicken in a 13 x 9-inch baking dish and bake until almost fully cooked, about 30 minutes.

2. Pour the pasta sauce over the chicken and top with the mozzarella; return the dish to the oven and bake until the chicken is cooked through and the cheese is melted.

3. Serve with the pasta and a salad on the side.

Caesar Salad

Order a Caesar salad at most restaurants and you'll get a high-calorie, high-fat disaster. This satisfying, healthy version can be served alone or topped with chicken for added protein.

MAKES 4 SERVINGS ■ EACH SERVING (1½ CUPS SALAD WITH MIXINGS) = 1 GREEN ;
1 TABLESPOON DRESSING = 1 GREEN ●; 2 OUNCES CHICKEN BREAST = 1 GREEN ●

PREP TIME: 15 minutes

COOK TIME: 5 minutes

READY TIME: 20 minutes

8 cups chopped romaine lettuce

¼ cup shredded Parmesan cheese

¾ cup whole wheat croutons, pita chips, or toasted baguette slices

8 ounces precooked chicken breast, cut into chunks (optional)

DRESSING

2 tablespoons fat-free mayonnaise

2 tablespoons olive oil

½ teaspoon minced garlic (about 1 clove)

Juice of ½ lemon (about 2 tablespoons)

1 teaspoon Worcestershire sauce

½ teaspoon anchovy paste (optional)

1. In a large bowl, combine the lettuce, cheese, and croutons or bread pieces.

2. In a small bowl, whisk together all the dressing ingredients.

3. Pour the dressing over the salad and toss before serving. Top with the chicken chunks, if desired.

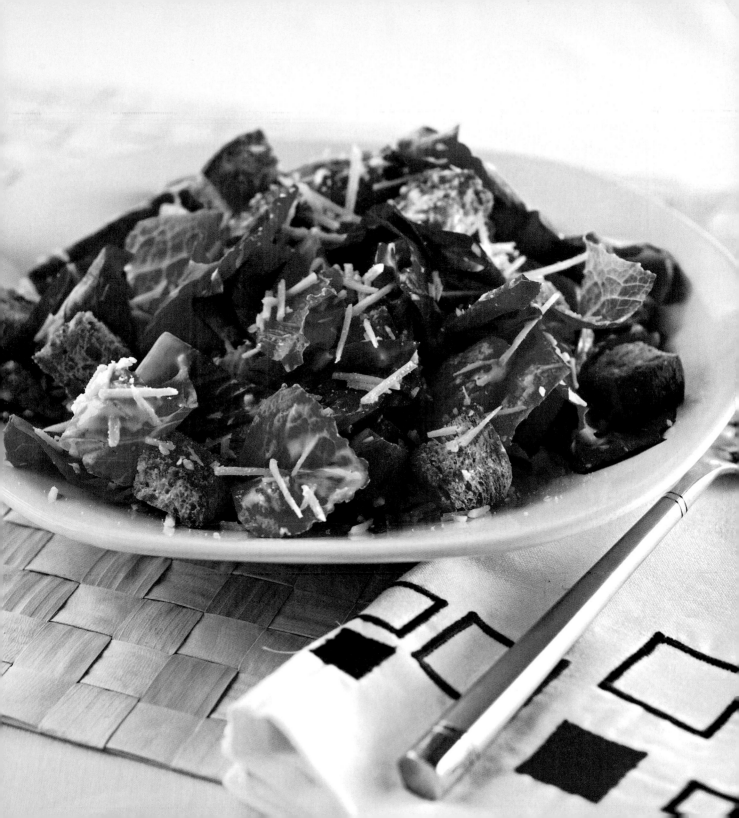

Weeknight Desserts

Many children like to have a little dessert after dinner. The best dessert is a healthy one. My kids love it when I sauté a banana in a skillet coated with vegetable cooking spray until it starts to caramelize and soften. It's delicious, and it's a **Free Fuel** dessert. My kids call it "Mommy Bananas."

If your kids must eat a dessert that's not a **Free Fuel**, they can take one of their **Green Light** foods from a meal or snack and use it for dessert. Or if they like to have something sweet every night, convert their two weekly **Red Light** foods into eight **Green Light** foods and have dessert every night.

Frosty Strawberry Yogurt Cupcakes

These cool treats are an easy make-ahead dessert—full of calcium, vitamin C, and protein.

MAKES 12 CUPCAKES ■ EACH SERVING (2 CUPCAKES) = 1 GREEN

PREP TIME: 5 minutes
FREEZE TIME: 2–3 hours
READY TIME: 2–3 hours

1 cup plain low-fat yogurt

10 ounces frozen strawberries, thawed

1 cup applesauce

1. Line the cups of a muffin pan with waxed baking liners (the kind used for cupcakes).

2. In a medium bowl, combine all the ingredients.

3. Pour the batter into individual baking liners.

4. Put the muffin pan in the freezer for approximately 2 to 3 hours until the mixture is firm, then serve.

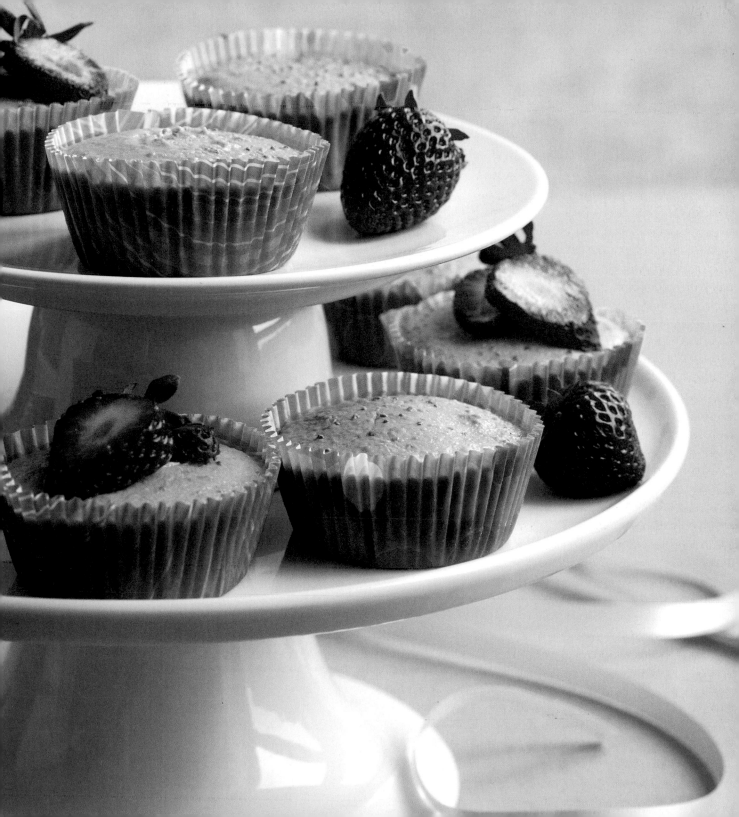

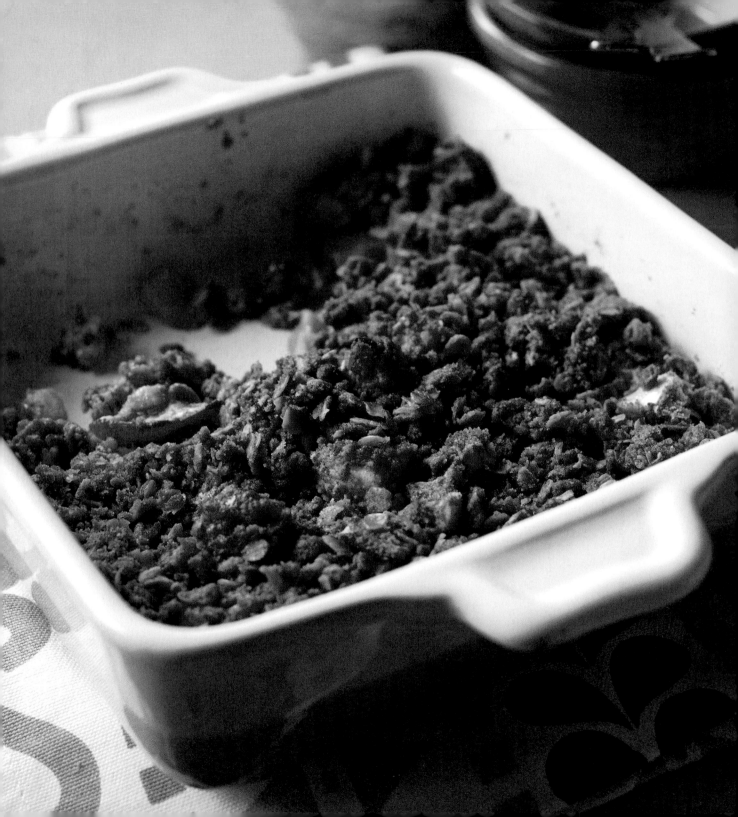

Apple Crisp

This recipe is comfort food at its best—but without all the calories. It's especially delicious when served warm. You can replace the apples with pears, peaches, plums, apricots, or whatever fruit is in season. If you are using a smaller-size fruit, double the amount of sliced fruit in the recipe.

MAKES 8 SERVINGS ■ EACH SERVING (2½ X 4-INCH PIECE) = 1 GREEN

PREP TIME: 10 minutes
COOK TIME: 35 minutes
READY TIME: 45 minutes

4 apples (I use Golden Delicious), peeled and cored

¼ cup brown sugar

½ cup whole wheat flour

½ cup rolled oats

2 tablespoons olive oil spread

2½ tablespoons cinnamon

Vegetable cooking spray

1 tablespoon honey

1. Preheat the oven to 375°F.

2. Dice the apples and put them in the bottom of an 8 x 8-inch baking dish.

3. Mix the remaining ingredients, except for the cooking spray and honey. Be sure to incorporate the olive oil spread thoroughly.

4. Spread the topping mixture on the apples.

5. Spray with cooking spray and drizzle with the honey.

6. Bake for 35 minutes.

8

● ● ●

WEIGHTY ZONE: SPECIAL OCCASIONS

Tempting high-fat, high-calorie dishes are the common denominator of birthdays, holidays, and other celebrations. For your kids, filling up on goodies can be a dream come true. But for you, these celebrations can be filled with concerns about how to keep your kids on their game plans without taking all the fun out of the event. Let's look at some strategies for five typical special occasions.

Special Occasion 1: Birthday Parties

Do you ever send your children off to school wondering if a classmate's birthday will be celebrated with homemade treats? Do you worry that your kids will feel left out if they can't have the sweets brought into the classroom? The truth is, they *are* likely to feel left out if they aren't able to join in a class birthday celebration. But your children don't need to say no to sweets! If sweets are saved for special occasions and are not part of their everyday diet, there's no reason why your kids can't enjoy a treat. Here are some guidelines to help you and your child navigate birthday parties.

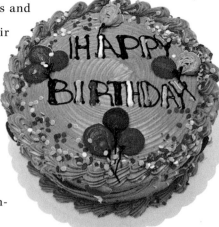

- If you're worried your child will overeat at a class party, be sure to talk to the teacher about your concerns. The teacher can hand out one cupcake, or three doughnut holes, or whatever the appropriate serving size is to each student and pack the rest away for the birthday boy or girl to take home.

- When it's your child's turn for a class birthday celebration, make healthy versions of your son's or daughter's favorite treat (such as the GREEN LIGHT CHOCOLATE CHIP BROWNIES, page 64), or simply pick up miniature versions of sweets, like Halloween-size candy bars or minicupcakes. Bring only enough servings so that each student in class (and the teacher!) can have an appropriate portion.

- If you're hosting a birthday party for your child at home, don't let food be the focus of the celebration. Plan games, organize outdoor activities, and play music. Instead of giving bags of candy to guests, create non-food goodie bags filled with small toys, whistles, stickers, colorful pens and pencils, and so forth.

- When it comes to birthday cake, if you don't have time to make a healthy cake yourself, pick up an ice-cream cake at the store. You may be surprised to learn that most ice-cream cakes (one slice = **Yellow** + **Green**) are actually better options for kids than bakery cakes (one slice = **Red** + **Yellow**). Consult the Appendix at the back of this book for suggestions.

- If you host a party somewhere other than your house, like a roller rink or a bowling alley, plan the menu in advance and see if the venue will allow you to bring your own food. Or better yet, throw the party at a park or outdoor recreation center where the kids can run around and get plenty of exercise!

- When your children are invited to parties held at fast-food restaurants, encourage them to make Green Light choices. Many franchises now offer healthier kids' menus. Suggest that youngsters opt for water instead of soda, choose fruit over french fries, and order a small hamburger without cheese instead of fried chicken nuggets.

- If you know about a party in advance, never send your child on an empty stomach. Make sure she eats lunch, dinner, or a snack (like a piece of fruit and a granola bar) before attending a party. She'll be less tempted to overeat if she's not hungry. When she gets to the party, encourage her to make only one trip to the snack table and pick one or two Red Light foods, depending on how many she has left for the week. If she does go off track, plan accordingly for a setback and be supportive.

Special Occasion 2: Halloween

For kids, Halloween is a highly anticipated event. According to the US Census Bureau, 36 million children ages 5 to 13 go trick-or-treating each year. Children love to plan elaborate costumes, get dressed up, play games, and—of course—eat Halloween treats. Halloween can be a lot of fun for the whole family, but it can also present a major roadblock for your children's game plans.

One of my most challenging cases involved the Martindales, a family of three, all of whom were obese. At 8 years old, son Josh weighed 115 pounds. His clothes were uncomfortably tight, and his energy was low. He just kept getting heavier and heavier—as did his parents. Josh just wasn't a happy kid.

The Martindales loved Halloween—and Halloween candy. I advised them to indulge (moderately) on the actual holiday but to get rid of all remaining candy the next day. Leftover Halloween candy can have a bigger impact on weight than you might think. Eating just two 75-calorie pieces of Halloween candy every day for 2 weeks adds up to 2,100 extra calories, or more than a half pound of fat!

But the Martindales just couldn't bear to part with their candy, and they all gained weight the week of Halloween. Josh's dad told me, "You don't understand. I can't throw the candy out. Josh really wants it." I persisted, explaining that parents should control children's eating and set the rules, especially when health is at stake. "Being an obese child increases the odds of serious health problems down the road," I reminded both parents.

After some initial grumbling, Dad and Mom got rid of the candy. To their surprise, Josh didn't throw a tantrum; he accepted their decision. They continued to stick to their game plans, and 4 months later, the Martindales had lost weight (and several clothing sizes). Josh is a happier kid with more energy, and life has been transformed in their household.

While Halloween can be a weak spot for many families, it's not necessary to forbid candy altogether. Like any treat, candy is fine in moderation, as long the other days of the month are filled with healthy foods. Here are some strategies for a happier, healthier Halloween:

- Feed your children nutritious food throughout the day and make sure you give them a snack or meal immediately before going trick-or-treating. If they "save up" all of their traffic lights and go trick-or-treating while they are ravenous, they are sure to overindulge.

- Offer to organize a Halloween parade for the little ghosts and goblins in your neighborhood so they can show off their costumes. Or sign up the family for a Halloween 5-K walk or run to burn off some of those candy calories!

- Throw a spooky party that includes fun Halloween games like "Pin the Eyes on the Witch," a three-legged monster race, or bobbing for apples—a healthy treat! Autumn is apple season, and apples are a great source of fiber and nutrients. Just don't coat them in caramel and sugar.

- Get all of the kids and their friends together to carve, decorate, or paint pumpkins. This takes the focus off the food and lets kids have loads of fun.

- Whip up a batch of healthy Halloween treats like Jell-O ghosts (made with sugar-free Jell-O and Halloween cookie cutters), roasted pumpkin seeds, or LOW-FAT PUMPKIN MUFFINS (page 181).

- When it comes to giving candy to trick-or-treaters, practice what you preach at home! Choose better treats, like 100-calorie packs, packets of microwave popcorn, or cereal bars. Or opt for non-food treats, like stickers, erasers, or glow-in-the-dark rings and bracelets. Not only will you be giving the neighborhood kids a healthier treat, but leftovers won't be a problem for your family.

- When your kids return home from trick-or-treating, indulge them a little. After all, it is Halloween, and they're kids! Give them a limit, and let them pick what they want to eat for the night. Each fun-size candy bar is one **Green,** which means your kids can exchange their two **Red Light** foods for eight fun-size candy bars to eat during the week. Let them eat some on Halloween night and then distribute the rest throughout the week. Throw out all other leftovers immediately to avoid further temptations!

- Be safe. Always check the collected items before allowing children to eat them.

Special Occasion 3: Traditional Holidays

The fall and early winter include the traditional celebrations of Rosh Hashanah, Thanksgiving, Hanukkah, and Christmas—when sweets and feasts abound. You don't have to be a party pooper when it comes to the holidays. Let your kids participate and have some goodies, within limits. Here are the strategies I recommend.

● Bring a healthy Green Light dish to events and celebrations. It's often difficult to find a healthy option when you eat at someone else's house. Prepare something your family likes so you know there will be something for them to eat. Your host and hostess will appreciate your generosity!

● Skip the big, fancy dinner plates and serve holiday meals on smaller, salad-size plates. If you are eating buffet-style, use dessert-size plates, which encourage smaller portions of the variety of available foods. Studies have shown that people who eat from smaller plates eat less food.

● Ease off on seconds. Be sure your children eat reasonable portions, and fill their plates only once. If they are still hungry after finishing their plate, offer filling low-calorie foods such as shrimp cocktail, vegetables, or fruit salad.

● Encourage your family to get up from the table immediately after the meal. It's tempting to take a few extra nibbles when the food is right in front of you. Take a walk or organize games in another room to help decrease the likelihood of mindless grazing.

● Pick one indulgence. Explain to your kids that they can choose one food they look forward to at that holiday every year, whether it's a dessert or main dish, and enjoy it. By choosing an indulgence, they won't feel deprived of holiday treats. One indulgence will not cause weight gain. Just be sure to monitor other unhealthy foods.

● Have sugarless gum on hand. Offer a stick to your kids if they crave something sweet after a meal and they don't have any Red Lights left that week. Chewing gum keeps their mouths occupied, and kids will be less likely to nibble on extra servings.

● Get moving. Encourage your family to stay active during the holiday season. Burning extra calories can make all the difference when it comes to weight management. Make every effort to exercise or engage in sports as a family. Instead of watching football on TV, have a scrimmage in your backyard! My family has an annual Thanksgiving football game, and everyone plays. We really enjoy it.

● Stay hydrated. Make sure there's plenty of water around so kids can sip a glass during and between meals, instead of snacking. Avoiding high-calorie beverages like punch, hot chocolate, apple cider, and eggnog during the holidays will circumvent extra calories, which do add up quickly.

Special Occasion 4: Valentine's Day

Many kids equate receiving chocolates on Valentine's Day with love. So how do you say "I love you" to the child you adore without going overboard on chocolate? In my family, we try to make the holiday more about expressing our feelings and less about candy. For example, we make our own homemade Valentines with construction paper, glue, markers, and glitter. It's a fun family activity. And when possible, I walk with my kids to personally deliver the cards to their friends in the neighborhood. Here are some additional suggestions.

- If you feel that Valentine's Day just isn't a holiday without chocolate, choose one small chocolate treat—such as a chocolate lollipop—or buy sugar-free chocolates.
- Talk to your children about their *real* hearts. Remind them that this organ needs special care to stay healthy and allow them to enjoy many more Valentine's Days. Eating nutritious food like fruits, veggies, and nuts keeps the heart healthy.
- Give a noncandy Valentine's Day gift like a new DVD, a book, a stuffed animal, or a game. Little girls love gifts like heart-shaped earrings, pink and red nail polish, and sparkly lip gloss. These gifts will make their day special without adding pounds.
- Remind kids that the true meaning of Valentine's Day is love! One of the most inspiring children I've ever met through my practice was 10-year-old Jamie, who had done very well on her game plan. She had lost 15 pounds and wanted to keep it off. On Valentine's Day, Jamie loved getting cards from friends—and also chocolate. But on this particular Valentine's Day, she was determined to remain on track with her game plan. So she told her friends and her parents that she would donate any candy she received to a charity for sick children. And that's exactly what she did. Teaching children to give back to others can be an eye-opening experience for young people and gives them a feeling of gratitude for what they have.

Special Occasion 5: Passover and Easter

Like most traditional holidays, Passover and Easter are filled with fattening food. High-calorie Passover foods include matzo brei, macaroons, brisket, matzo kugel, roasted potatoes, dried fruit compote, and a myriad of sweets. Easter includes caloric food traditions such as baskets of Easter eggs and candy, hot cross buns, honey pastries, carrot cake, and glazed ham.

Whatever our traditions, we all face the same problems when it comes to being healthy during the holidays. Here are some tips to handle these food fests.

- Think small sizes. Allow your kids to taste a small amount of each dish served. By limiting portion sizes, children can try lots of different foods they probably don't have an opportunity to eat the rest of the year.
- Bring fruit for dessert. After indulging in a special holiday meal, limit dessert calories. Bring your hostess a fruit platter for dessert (even if you aren't asked) so you can ensure a healthy dessert option for you and your family.
- Don't let your kids waste calories on foods they can eat anytime. Have them save calorie indulgences for the special foods eaten for the holiday. Eat a Cadbury egg instead of a brownie. Skip the mashed potatoes and serve a small portion of matzo kugel instead.
- As you would on Halloween and Valentine's Day, monitor how much Easter candy your child eats. Especially if your children are on weight-loss

game plans, consider filling their Easter baskets with books and stuffed bunnies or low-calorie treats like cereal bars, small boxes of raisins, or pieces of whole fruit.

- Get creative in the kitchen. Modify unhealthy and fattening dishes to a lower-fat, lower-calorie recipe while keeping the flavor. LOW-FAT EASTER CARROT CAKE (page 173) and POTATO KUGEL (page 170), for example, are healthier versions of traditional recipes. Revamp family favorites by replacing whole milk or cream with fat-free half-and-half; substitute half of the shortening, butter, or oil in a recipe with applesauce or prune puree (you may need to reduce baking time by 25 percent); replace whole-fat cheese with reduced-fat or fat-free cheese; or trade whipping cream for evaporated skim milk or fat-free whipped topping. The possibilities are endless.

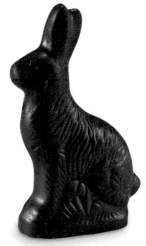

Holiday Recipes

Here are several mouthwatering holiday favorites that your family can enjoy without overindulging. Remember—portion control is key!

Holiday Ham

This holiday favorite can be healthier than many people realize. Just be sure to choose a lean ham and trim away excess fat.

MAKES 18 SERVINGS ■ EACH SERVING (2 OUNCES) = 1 YELLOW

PREP TIME: 10 minutes
COOK TIME: 1 hour 5 minutes
READY TIME: 1 hour 30 minutes

5½–6 pound 33 percent less-sodium smoked, fully cooked ham half
Vegetable cooking spray
½ cup red pepper jelly
½ cup pineapple preserves
¼ cup packed brown sugar
¼ teaspoon ground cloves

1. Preheat the oven to 425°F.

2. Trim the fat and rind from the ham. Score the outside of the ham in a diamond pattern.

3. Place the ham on a broiler pan coated with vegetable cooking spray.

4. Combine the jelly, preserves, brown sugar, and cloves, stirring with a whisk until well blended. Brush about a third of the jelly mixture over the ham.

5. Bake for 5 minutes.

6. Reduce the oven temperature to 325°F (do not remove the ham from the oven), and bake for an additional 45 minutes, basting the ham with the jelly mixture every 15 minutes.

7. Transfer the ham to a serving platter, and let stand 15 minutes before slicing.

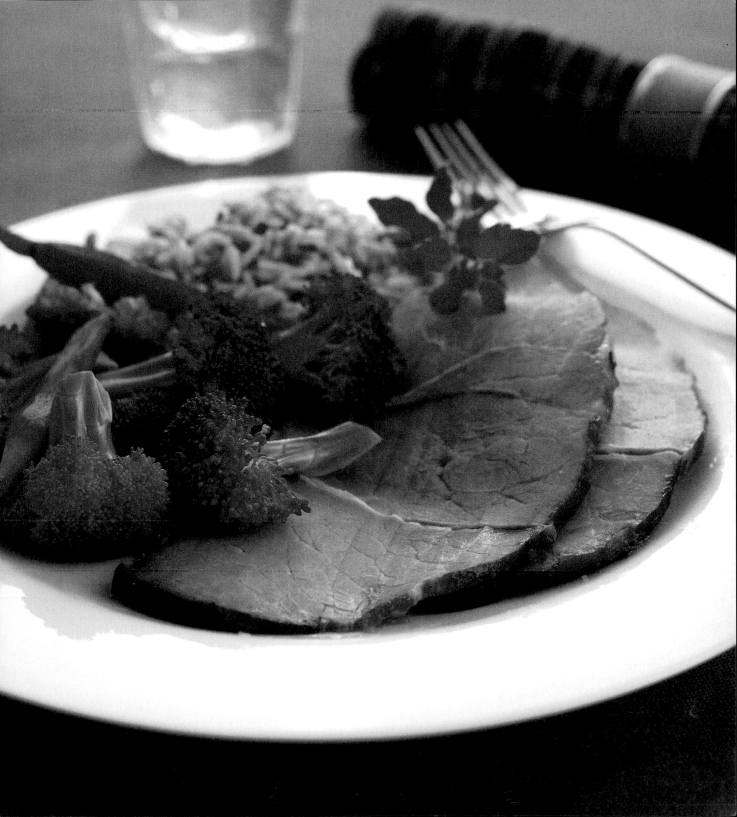

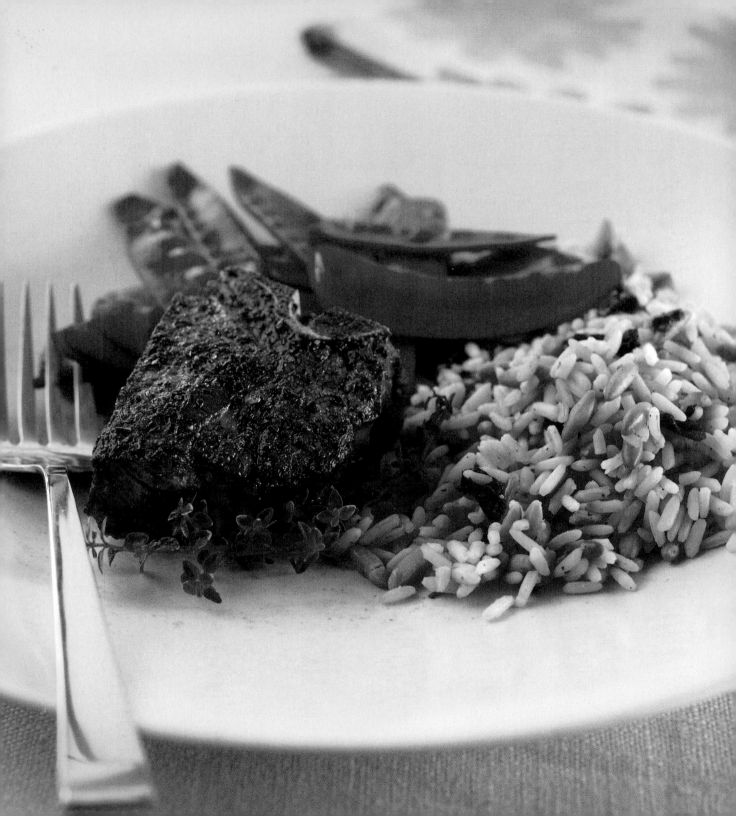

Lemon and Herb Lamb Chops

Lamb doesn't have to be a challenge to prepare. Here's a quick, nutritious way to cook lamb chops that both grown-ups and kids love.

MAKES 4 SERVINGS ■ EACH SERVING (1 CHOP) = 1 YELLOW ● + 1 GREEN ●

PREP TIME: 20 minutes

COOK TIME: 10 minutes

READY TIME: 30 minutes

4 lamb loin chops (4½ ounces each)

¼ cup lemon juice

1 teaspoon dried oregano

1 teaspoon dried thyme

1 teaspoon ground black pepper

Pinch of salt

Olive oil cooking spray

1. Trim the chops of all visible fat.

2. Place the chops in a glass baking dish with the lemon juice, oregano, thyme, black pepper, and salt. Turn to coat, then marinate for 15 minutes.

3. Coat a heavy nonstick skillet with cooking spray. Cook the chops over medium-high heat for 4 to 5 minutes on each side, depending on the thickness and desired doneness.

Spinach and Mushroom Bake

Free Fuel galore—that's what you'll serve up here. The variety of veggies in this dish supplies a variety of nutrients.

MAKES 9 SERVINGS ■ EACH SERVING (2½ X 4-INCH PIECE) = 1 GREEN

PREP TIME: 15 minutes
COOK TIME: 45 minutes–1 hour
READY TIME: 1 hour 15 minutes

Canola cooking spray

1 cup chopped onion

2 cups sliced mushrooms

2 cups grated or diced carrots

1 cup diced zucchini

2 (10-ounce) boxes frozen, chopped spinach, thawed and gently squeezed to eliminate excess water

½ cup matzo meal

3 large eggs, lightly beaten

¾ cup egg substitute

¼ teaspoon salt

¼ teaspoon ground black pepper

2 teaspoons low-sodium chicken broth powder

1. Preheat the oven to 325°F. Coat a 9 x 9-inch or an 8 x 8-inch baking pan with cooking spray.

2. Coat a large nonstick skillet with cooking spray. Add the onion and mushrooms, cover the pan, and cook over medium heat, stirring occasionally, until the mushrooms are lightly browned.

3. Transfer the mushroom mixture to a large bowl and add the remaining ingredients. Mix thoroughly.

4. Spread the mixture into the prepared pan and bake for 45 to 60 minutes, until firm and lightly browned on the bottom.

Maple Roasted Sweet Potatoes

There's nothing more delicious than making sweet potatoes a little sweeter, especially with the addition of maple syrup. This side dish is the perfect complement to baked ham.

MAKES 12 SERVINGS ■ EACH SERVING (4 OUNCES) = 1 GREEN

PREP TIME: 20 minutes
COOK TIME: 1 hour–1 hour
             5 minutes
READY TIME: 1½ hours

2½ pounds sweet potatoes, peeled and cut into 1½-inch pieces

⅓ cup pure maple syrup

2 tablespoons butter, melted

1½ tablespoons lemon juice

½ teaspoon salt

½ teaspoon ground black pepper

1. Preheat the oven to 400°F.

2. Arrange the sweet potatoes in an even layer in a 9 x 13-inch glass baking dish.

3. In a small bowl, combine the syrup, butter, lemon juice, salt, and pepper.

4. Pour the mixture over the sweet potatoes and toss to coat.

5. Cover and bake the sweet potatoes for 15 minutes.

6. Uncover the dish and stir. Continue to bake the potatoes, stirring every 15 minutes, until tender and starting to brown, about 45 to 50 minutes.

Roasted Garlic Potatoes

This delicious side dish pairs potatoes and garlic—a yummy, healthy combination.

MAKES 12 SERVINGS ■ EACH SERVING (4 OUNCES) = 1 GREEN

PREP TIME: 10 minutes
COOK TIME: 1 hour 30 minutes
READY TIME: 1 hour 40 minutes

9 potatoes (about 4 ounces each), sliced

1 teaspoon salt

2 teaspoons dried dill

1 whole garlic bulb

3 tablespoons reduced-calorie margarine, melted

1. Preheat the oven to 350°F.

2. Combine all the ingredients in a large bowl, tossing to coat the potatoes well.

3. Pour the mixture into a 13 × 9-inch baking dish. Use a scraper to scrape all the margarine and seasonings from the sides of the bowl, drizzling the last bits over the potatoes in the dish.

4. Bake for about 1½ hours or until the potatoes are cooked through and lightly browned.

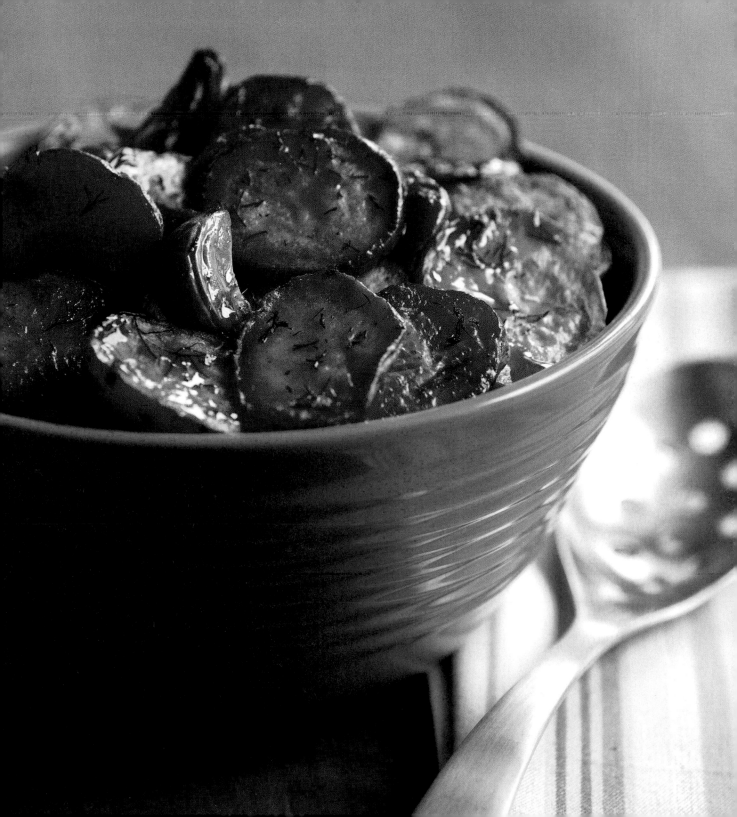

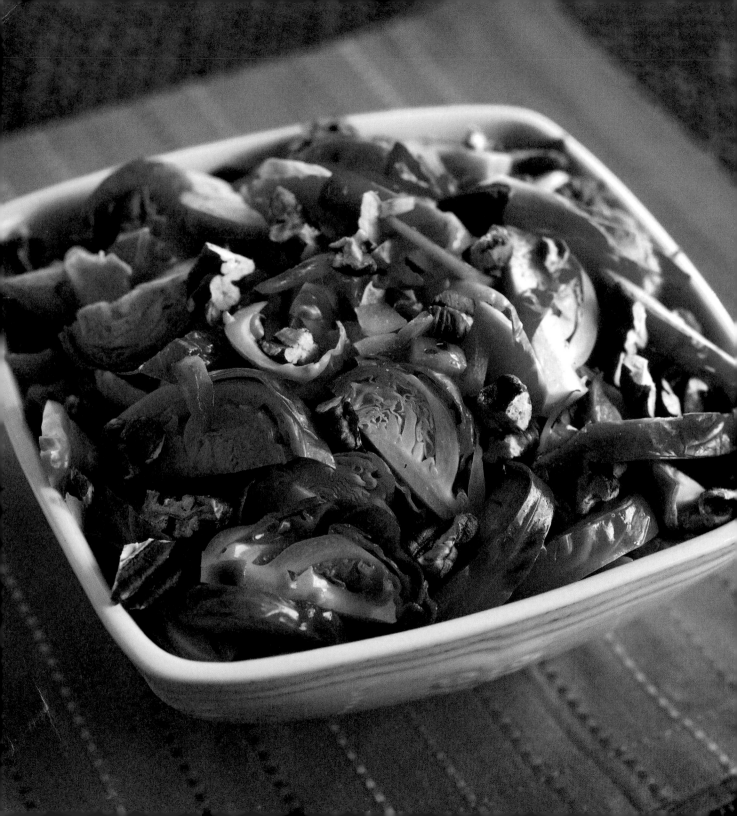

Brussels Sprouts with Pecans

Sometimes it's hard to get kids to eat brussels sprouts, but prepare them with pecans and you'll hardly have a battle!

MAKES 8 SERVINGS ■ 1 SERVING (⅔ CUP) = 1 GREEN

PREP TIME: 5 minutes

COOK TIME: 11 minutes

READY TIME: 16 minutes

2 teaspoons butter

1 cup chopped onion

4 garlic cloves, thinly sliced

8 cups halved and thinly sliced brussels sprouts (about 1½ pounds)

½ cup fat-free, reduced-sodium chicken broth

1 tablespoon sugar

½ teaspoon salt

8 teaspoons coarsely chopped pecans, toasted

1. Melt the butter in a large nonstick skillet over medium-high heat.

2. Add the onion and garlic and sauté for 4 minutes or until lightly browned.

3. Stir in the brussels sprouts and sauté for 2 minutes.

4. Add the broth and sugar and cook, stirring frequently, for 5 minutes or until the liquid almost evaporates. Stir in the salt.

5. Sprinkle with the pecans.

Ham and Fruit Salad

What I love about this salad is that it uses figs. Figs are very high in fiber, and they are delicious. This is a super-food salad.

MAKES 4 SERVINGS ■ EACH SERVING: 4 SLICES OF HAM = 1 GREEN
MIXED GREENS AND FRUIT = FREE FUEL; 1 TABLESPOON DRESSING = 1 GREEN

PREP TIME: 5 minutes
COOK TIME: None
READY TIME: 5 minutes

2 cups mixed field greens

½ cup diced cantaloupe

4 medium figs, quartered

2 tablespoons diced red onion

8 slices smoked deli ham, cut in strips

DRESSING
2 teaspoons olive oil

1 teaspoon balsamic vinegar

⅛ teaspoon ground black pepper

1. Prepare salad ingredients in a large bowl and place to the side.

2. In a small mixing bowl, whisk the olive oil slowly into the vinegar. Add the pepper.

3. Pour the dressing over the salad and serve.

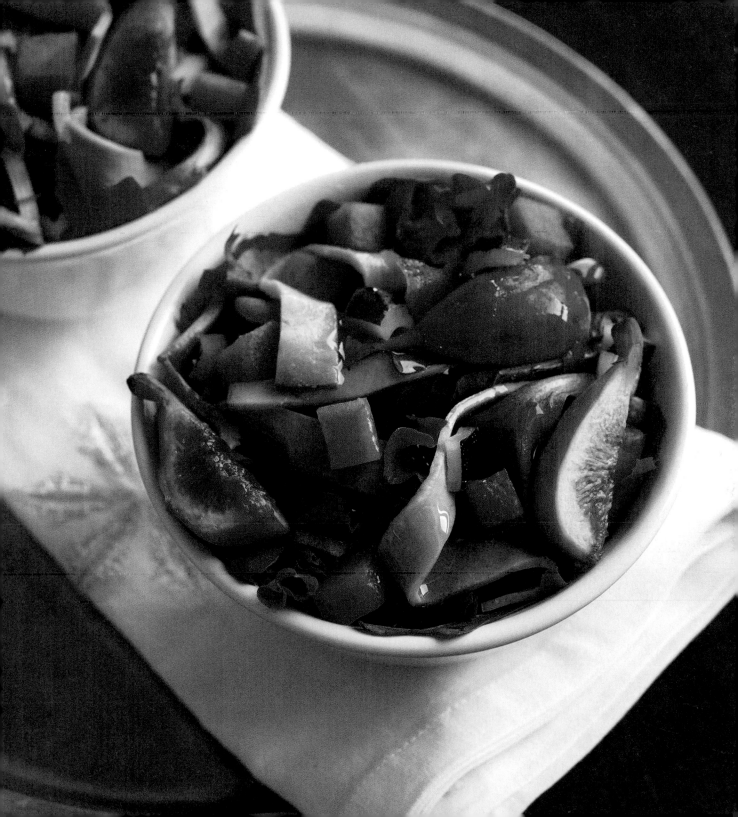

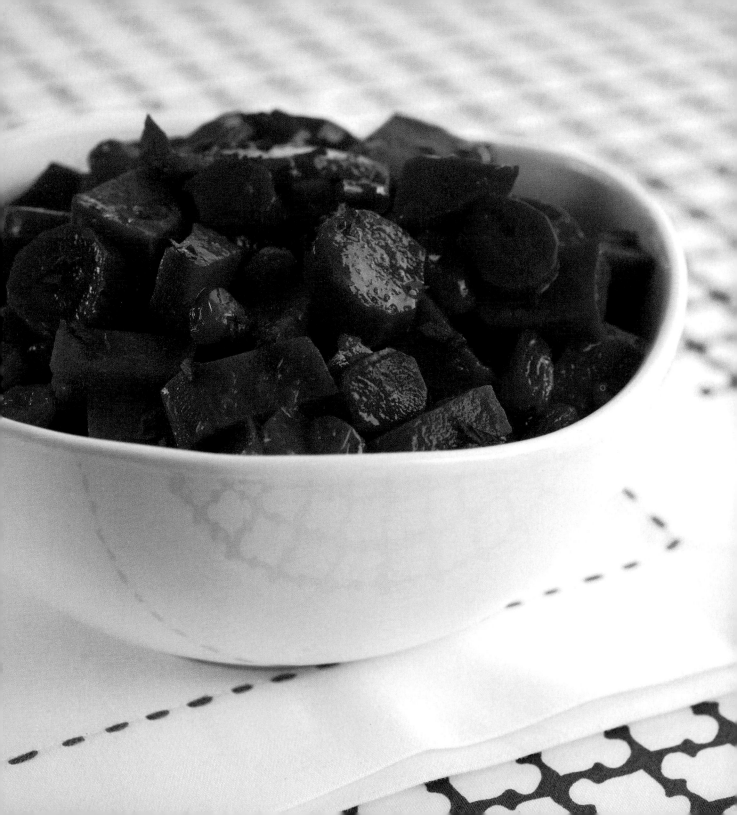

Carrot Tzimmes

Here's a traditional favorite that is loaded with beta-carotene, an important health-building anti-oxidant. The natural sweetness of this dish will make everyone want seconds—so watch your portions!

MAKES 6 SERVINGS ■ 1 SERVING (¾ CUP) = 1 YELLOW

PREP TIME: 10 minutes
COOK TIME: 30 minutes
READY TIME: 40 minutes

1 pound carrots, peeled and
    sliced into coins

5 large sweet potatoes, peeled
    and quartered

1 tablespoon canola oil

1½ tablespoons honey

1½ tablespoons brown sugar

4 tablespoons freshly squeezed
    orange juice

⅓ cup seedless golden raisins or
    ½ cup pitted prunes

Kosher salt and ground black
    pepper to taste

Minced fresh parsley

1. Mix everything except the parsley together in a medium saucepan and bring to a boil over high heat. Cover, reduce the heat, and simmer gently for about 25 minutes, until the carrots are crisp tender and the potatoes are tender but firm.

2. Remove the cover from the pan, raise the heat, and cook the carrots until most of the liquid has evaporated and the sauce is thickened, about 5 minutes.

3. Sprinkle the parsley on top and serve.

Potato Kugel

Yummy is the best word to describe this version of the classic potato pancake. Use low-sodium chicken broth to cut the salt.

MAKES 8 SERVINGS ■ EACH SERVING (½ CUP) = 1 YELLOW

PREP TIME: 15 minutes
COOK TIME: 1 hour
READY TIME: 1 hour 15 minutes

1 large onion, grated

6 large potatoes, peeled and grated (about 1¾ pounds of potatoes before peeling)

2 eggs, well beaten

½ cup egg substitute, or 2–4 regular eggs

¼ cup canola oil

¼ cup condensed chicken broth or low-sodium chicken broth

Kosher salt and ground black pepper to taste

1. Preheat the oven to 400°F.

2. Grate the onion first. Grate the potatoes and add to the onion to stop the potatoes from turning brown. Further chop half of this mixture with the blade of the food processor. This makes the kugel less dense.

3. Mix the onions, potatoes, and the remaining ingredients together. Pour the mixture into a 2- or 3-quart rectangular baking dish.

4. Bake for about 60 minutes or until very brown and crusty.

5. Cut into squares to serve.

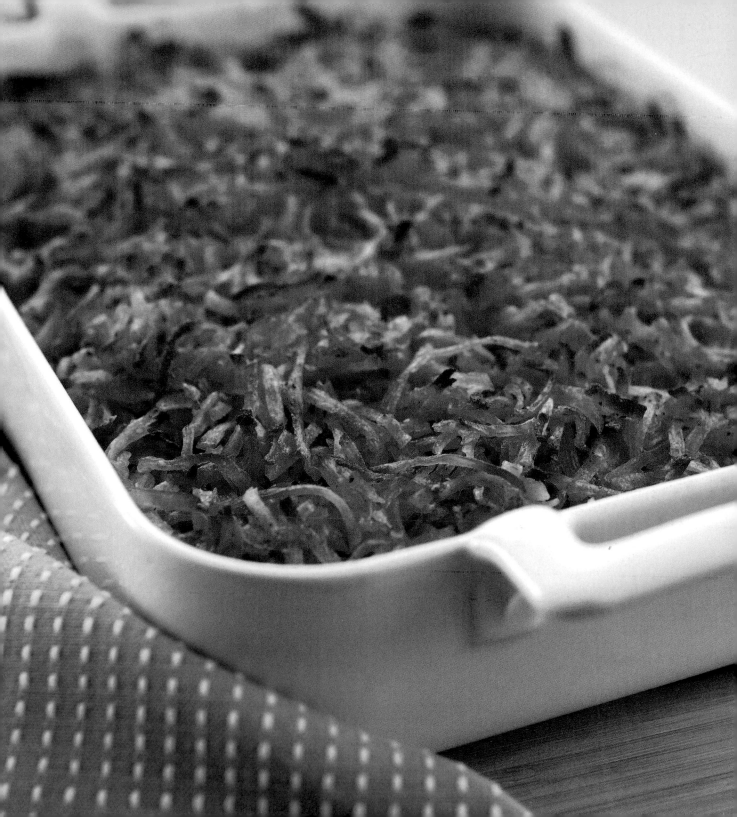

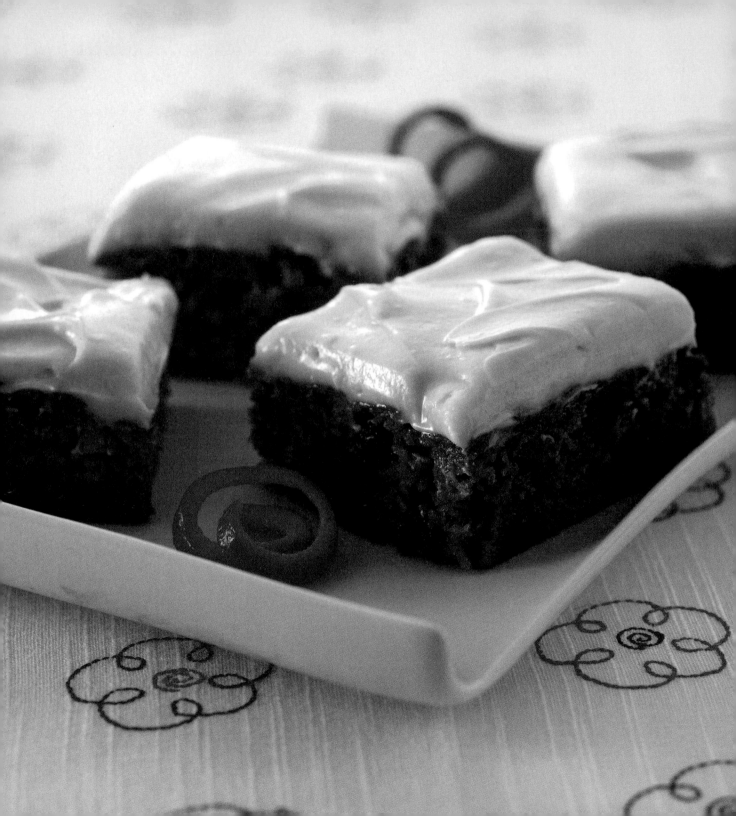

Low-Fat Easter Carrot Cake

To decrease the fat content in baked goods, try substituting applesauce or prune puree for butter or oil. This cake is made even more moist and flavorful by the addition of applesauce.

MAKES 20 SERVINGS ■ EACH SERVING (1 SQUARE) = 1 YELLOW

PREP TIME: 15 minutes
COOK TIME: 35–40 minutes
READY TIME: 1 hour 5 minutes

Nonstick, fat-free cooking spray

1 cup all-purpose flour

1 cup whole wheat flour

2 teaspoons baking soda

1 teaspoon ground cinnamon

½ teaspoon allspice

¼ teaspoon nutmeg

4 egg whites

1¼ cups packed brown sugar

1 cup unsweetened applesauce

½ cup low-fat buttermilk

1 teaspoon vanilla extract

1 (8-ounce) can crushed pineapple, drained

2 cups shredded carrots

½ cup raisins

¼ cup chopped walnuts

FROSTING

¼ cup light cream cheese

¼ cup fat-free cream cheese

1 teaspoon lemon juice

½ teaspoon vanilla extract

2 cups confectioners' sugar

1. Preheat the oven to 350°F. Spray a 13 x 9-inch baking pan with cooking spray.

2. In a large bowl, combine the flours, baking soda, cinnamon, allspice, and nutmeg and stir with a whisk.

3. In another bowl, beat the egg whites until soft peaks form. Beat in the sugar slowly, followed by the applesauce, buttermilk, and vanilla; add this to the flour mixture and stir until it is just moist. Stir in the pineapple, carrots, raisins, and walnuts.

4. Spoon the batter into the baking pan and bake for 35 to 40 minutes, until a toothpick inserted into the center comes out clean. Cool on a wire rack before frosting.

5. To make the frosting, beat the cream cheeses together with the lemon juice and vanilla. Add in the confectioners' sugar until you get the desired consistency.

6. Spread the frosting over the cooled cake and cut the cake into 20 squares.

Low-Fat Easter Angel Food Cake

Here's an even lighter version of a classic favorite. Try topping it with fresh, Free Fuel berries for extra nutrition and a beautiful presentation.

MAKES 20 SERVINGS ■ EACH SERVING (1 SLICE) = 1 GREEN

PREP TIME: 10 minutes
COOK TIME: 30–35 minutes
COOL TIME: 1 hour
READY TIME: 1 hour 45 minutes

1 cup cake flour

¾ cup + 2 tablespoons Splenda or other low-calorie sweetener

1½ teaspoons vanilla extract

½ teaspoon almond extract

12 large egg whites

1½ teaspoons cream of tartar

¼ teaspoon salt

¾ cup sugar

1. Preheat the oven to 375°F.

2. Sift together the cake flour and Splenda or sweetener and set aside.

3. Combine the extracts in a small bowl and set aside.

4. In a mixing bowl, beat the egg whites, cream of tartar, and salt until soft peaks form. Slowly add the sugar, then beat on high until stiff peaks form.

5. Beating on low, slowly add the flour mixture and extracts to the eggs. Make sure you fold in the batter from the sides and bottom of your mixing bowl.

6. Spoon the batter into an ungreased, two-piece angel food cake pan. Move a knife through the batter to remove air pockets.

7. Bake for 30 to 35 minutes or until the top springs back when touched lightly with your finger.

8. Cool upside down on a cooling rack for at least 1 hour before removing the cake from the pan. When the cake is cool, run a knife around the edge of the pan and invert on a plate.

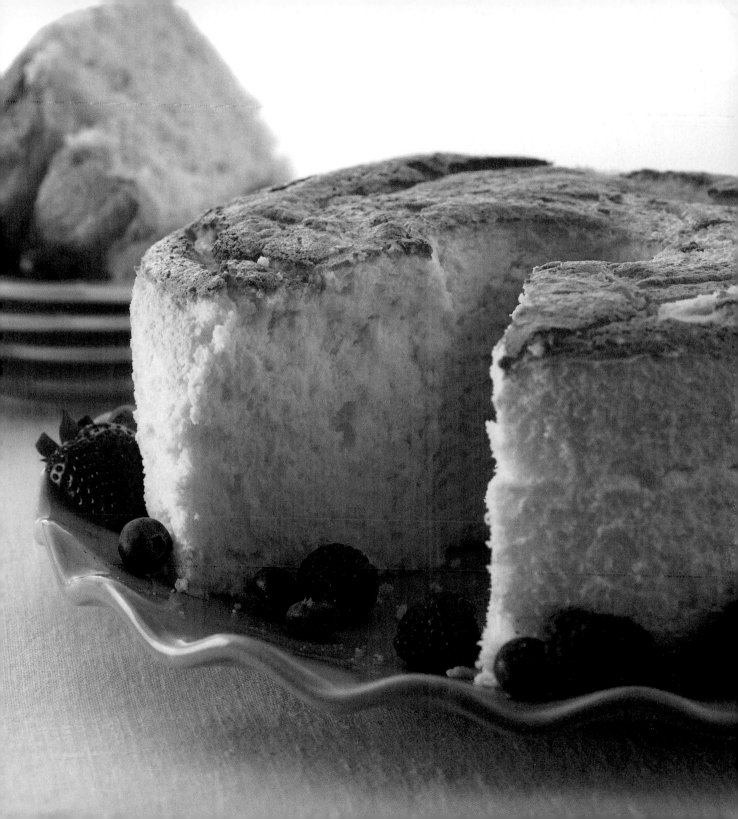

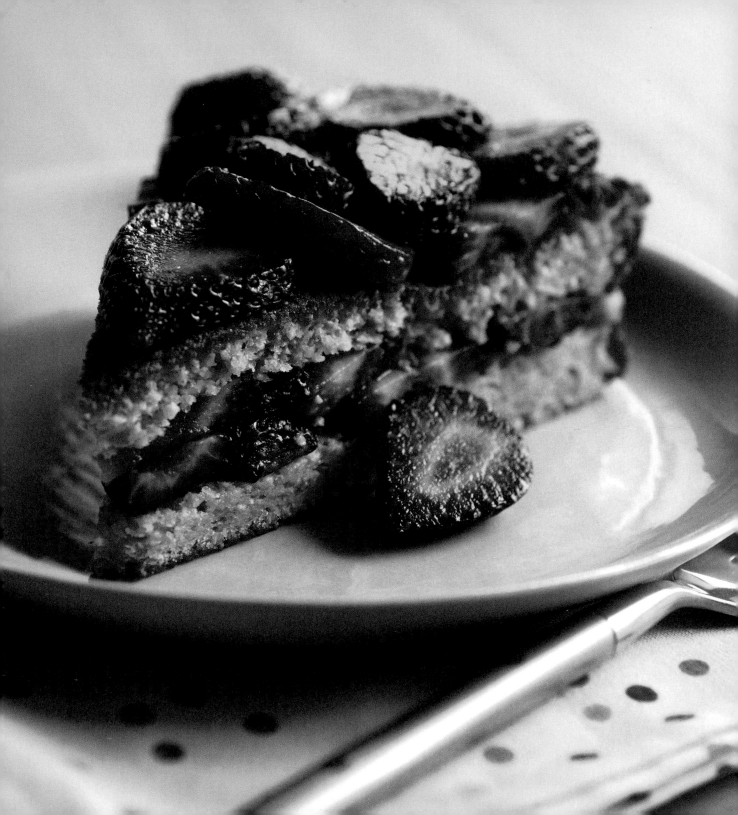

Matzo-Lemon Sponge Cake

Here's a fun, easy way to make sponge cake. It's low in fat and makes the perfect holiday dessert.

MAKES 12 SERVINGS ■ EACH SERVING (1 SLICE) = 1 YELLOW

PREP TIME: 10 minutes
COOK TIME: 45 minutes
READY TIME: 1 hour

8 egg whites
4 egg yolks
½ cup lemonade
1½ cups sugar
½ teaspoon salt
Juice and grated rind of 1 lemon
1 cup sifted matzo cake meal
Strawberries (optional)

1. Preheat the oven to 350°F. Line just the bottom of a 10-inch springform pan or the bottoms of 2 loaf pans with parchment or waxed paper.

2. Beat the egg whites until stiff and set aside.

3. Beat the egg yolks and lemonade until light. Add the sugar and beat for 1 minute. Add the salt, lemon juice and rind, and cake meal and beat on low until blended. On low speed, gently beat in the egg whites (or fold in with a spatula).

4. Once it's well mixed, pour the batter into the prepared pan(s) and bake until golden, about 45 minutes for the springform pan or around 20 minutes for the loaf pans.

5. Invert the pan until the cake is cool. Use a knife to cut around edges and remove the cake from the pan.

6. Cut the cake with a serrated knife into layers, if desired. Serve with strawberries between the layers, if using.

Light Honey Cake

My family loves this rich-tasting dessert and looks forward to it at holidays.

MAKES 12 SERVINGS ■ EACH SERVING (1 SLICE) = 1 YELLOW

PREP TIME: 10 minutes
COOK TIME: 1 hour 20 minutes
READY TIME: 1 hour 40 minutes

Vegetable cooking spray

1 tablespoon dry bread crumbs

¼ cup hot water

2 teaspoons instant espresso granules or 4 teaspoons instant coffee granules

½ cup sugar

2 large eggs

½ cup honey

3 tablespoons stick margarine, melted

1¾ cups all-purpose flour

1 teaspoon baking powder

1 teaspoon ground cinnamon

¼ teaspoon salt

½ cup chopped walnuts

½ cup golden raisins

1. Preheat the oven to 325°F. Coat an 8 x 4-inch loaf pan with cooking spray, then dust with the bread crumbs; set aside.

2. Combine the water and espresso or coffee granules in a small bowl; set aside.

3. In a medium bowl, combine the sugar and eggs and stir well with a whisk. Add the honey and margarine and stir well.

4. In another bowl, combine the flour, baking powder, cinnamon, and salt.

5. Add half of the flour mixture to the sugar mixture and stir well. Add the coffee mixture to the sugar mixture and stir well. Add the remaining flour mixture and stir just until the flour is moistened. Stir in the walnuts and raisins.

6. Spoon the batter into the prepared pan and bake for 1 hour and 20 minutes or until a wooden pick inserted in the center comes out clean.

7. Cool the cake in the pan on a wire rack for 10 minutes, then remove from the pan. Cool the cake completely on the wire rack. Cut into slices and serve.

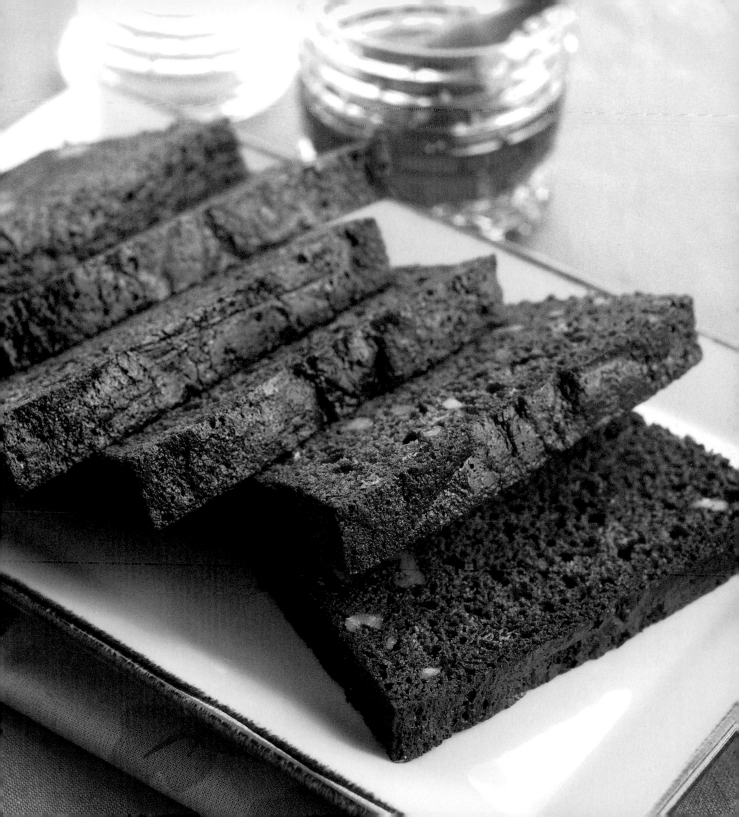

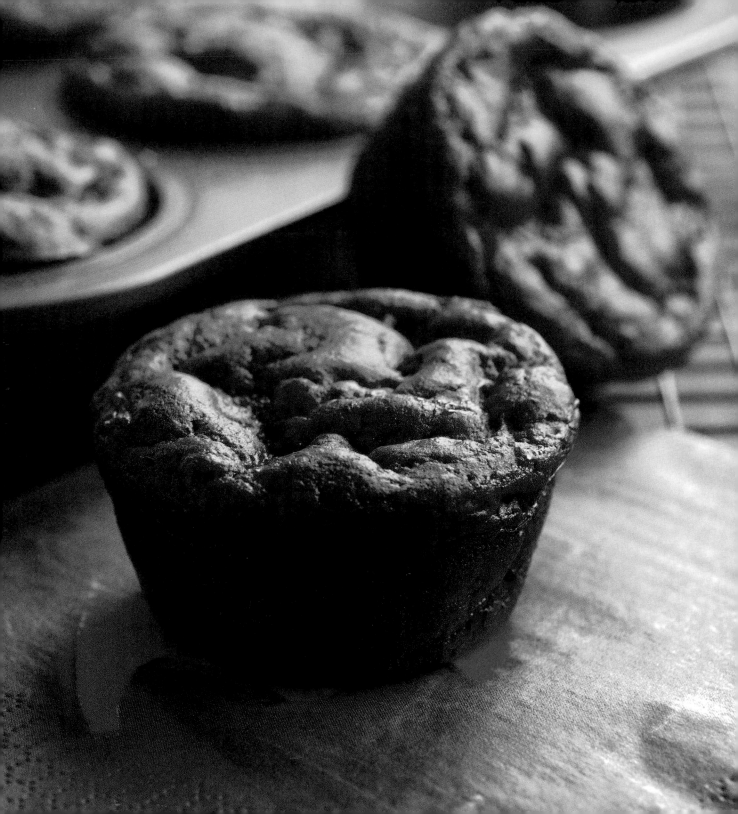

Low-Fat Pumpkin Muffins

What is Halloween without pumpkins? Here's a way to incorporate beta-carotene–rich pumpkin into a delicious Halloween muffin. There's nothing scary about these treats!

MAKES 6 SERVINGS ■ EACH SERVING (1 MUFFIN) = 1 YELLOW

PREP TIME: 10 minutes
COOK TIME: 20 minutes
READY TIME: 40 minutes

⅔ cup nonfat dry milk

¼ cup Splenda

6 tablespoons flour

1 teaspoon baking soda

2½ teaspoons pumpkin pie spice

1 teaspoon cinnamon

2 eggs

1 cup canned pumpkin

½ cup grated carrots

4 tablespoons raisins

1 teaspoon vanilla

1. Preheat the oven to 350°F.

2. Combine the dry milk, Splenda, flour, baking soda, pumpkin pie spice, and cinnamon in a bowl and sift.

3. Combine the eggs, pumpkin, carrots, raisins, and vanilla in a small bowl.

4. Add the dry ingredients to the wet ingredients slowly without overmixing.

5. Bake for 20 minutes.

6. Let cool in muffin tins for 5 minutes, then transfer to wire cooling rack to cool completely.

Green Light Christmas Thumbprint Cookies

Thumbprint cookies have become a Christmas tradition—they're sweetly satisfying and pretty enough to take to a party or serve to guests. Try this low-fat version when holiday cookie time rolls around.

MAKES 20 COOKIES ■ EACH SERVING (1 COOKIE) = 1 GREEN

PREP TIME: 15 minutes

COOK TIME: 10 minutes

READY TIME: 30 minutes

¼ cup low-fat butter, softened

½ cup light brown sugar, firmly packed

1 egg

1 teaspoon vanilla extract

1½ cups all-purpose flour

¼ teaspoon salt

½ cup good-quality raspberry jam (or strawberry, cherry, or any other red jam)

1. Preheat the oven to 350°F. Line a large baking sheet with parchment paper or a silicone mat.

2. In a large bowl, cream the butter and brown sugar together, using an electric mixer. Add the egg and vanilla and mix until blended.

3. Whisk together the flour and salt in a small bowl. Gradually add the flour mixture to the wet ingredients and mix with a wooden spoon, forming a large ball.

4. If the dough is sticky, refrigerate for an hour before proceeding. Otherwise, form 1-inch balls and place them 1 inch apart on the baking sheet, making a deep thumbprint in the center of each.

5. Bake for 10 minutes. Remove from the oven. After 1 minute, place the cookies on a wire rack to cool.

6. Add a dollop of jam to the center of each cookie. Let set for at least 1 hour before serving.

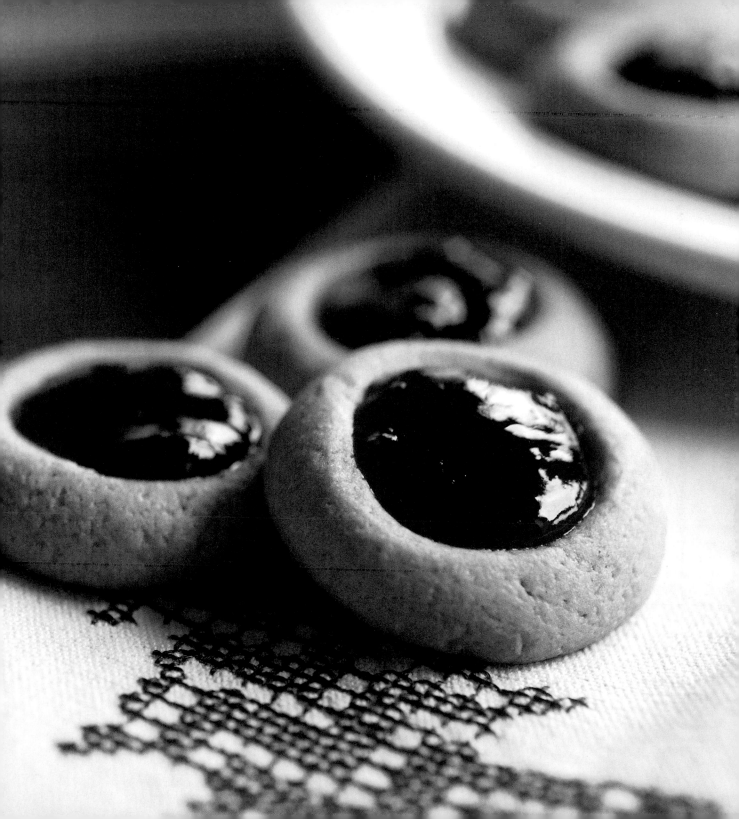

VACATION TIME

Vacations can present roadblocks to good nutrition. But don't despair! With a bit of planning, a few simple tools, and the willingness to spend some time seeking out foods that fit your game plan, your trip away won't trip you up. Here are some tips for healthy travel.

● Plan ahead. Either bring healthy snacks for the hotel room or, when you get to your destination, stop at a grocery or convenience store and pick some up. Examples include nuts, fruit, whole grain bread, and peanut butter.

● Pack healthy meals and snacks for the car or the airplane. If you plan to drive a long distance, make a healthy lunch or dinner at home, wrap it up, and pack it in a cooler. When the family is hungry, pull over to a rest stop to enjoy your healthy meal and stretch your legs. While in transit, encourage your kids to play games, listen to music, draw, or color to help pass the time instead of mindlessly grazing on snacks.

● Watch out for breakfast buffets. You can eat a day's worth of calories (or more) with just one trip through the line, so I recommend indulging in the breakfast buffet only on the last day of vacation. Pack cereal bars and fruit for the other days so that your family has healthy options, even if the hotel doesn't.

● Pay attention to portions. Many restaurant servings are huge—and research has proven that the more food that's put in front of someone, the more they will eat. When you walk into a new restaurant, look at the size of the meals on other customers' tables. If portions are huge, consider splitting dishes with someone else in the family.

● Be reasonable. Not all of your children's lower-calorie options will be available while you're out of town, so do the best you can. Don't let your child give up completely. If he or she says, "I'm on vacation this week so I'm going to eat whatever I want," pounds may pile on.

● Help everyone in your family stay active while on vacation. Walk, hike, bike, swim, or exercise in the hotel gym to burn calories.

Once all of these holidays and celebrations are said and done, it's important to refocus all family members on their game plans. Make sure that nutritious foods such as fruits and vegetables are available to your kids year-round. That way, you'll prepare them for a lifetime of responsible food choices, even during special occasions.

9
• • •

RESTAURANTS: BE PREPARED

Nothing makes a child feel more grown-up than going out to dinner. And for parents, dining out offers a convenient, fun escape from the stress of everyday meal preparation. Eating at restaurants has become a fixture of modern family life, and there's no sign of that changing anytime soon. But here's the catch: According to one large study published in the *Journal of Nutrition Education and Behavior* in 2002, kids (and their parents) eat up to 32 percent more calories while eating out than they do at home. Further, most of these restaurant meals are higher in total fat and saturated fat on a per-calorie basis and contain less fiber, calcium, and iron than food eaten at home. Of course, more calories equal more weight gain. Restaurants, with their large portions and high-

fat fare, contribute to the child obesity epidemic. That's why, ultimately, it's up to you as a parent to help your kids make healthy food choices outside the home and teach them that dining out can be a fun and healthy experience.

Steer Clear of Kids' Menus and Other Restaurant Traps!

In recent years, many fast-food restaurants have responded to demands for healthier choices for kids and adults. But at most sit-down restaurants, children's menus—with their familiar and cheap offerings—have lagged behind. With few exceptions, kids' menus are loaded with fat and calories in the form of foods such as chicken nuggets, hot dogs, cheeseburgers, pizza, and french fries. My husband and I have found that it's almost always better to skip the kids' menu altogether and either order our children's meals off of the regular menu or special order foods for them. Here are some additional tips for dining out with your kids.

- Before you leave the house, decide where you'd like to go. If possible, review the restaurant menu online before you head out.
- Talk about food options in advance so there are no arguments over the menu at the restaurant. Make sure your kids know which traffic lights they will be using and what kinds of foods they would like to eat with those lights.
- Learn how to decode menu descriptions. When scanning for healthy choices, look for the following terms: *grilled, steamed, garden fresh, broiled, baked, roasted, poached,* or *steamed.* Avoid choices that contain words like *deep-fried, pan-fried, basted, batter-dipped, breaded, cheesy, creamy,* or *crispy.*
- Don't be afraid to ask for modifications. If a dish comes with sour cream, ask for salsa instead. Switch out creamy Alfredo for red pasta sauce. And ask for mustard instead of mayonnaise on sandwiches.

- To control portion sizes, share an entrée or appetizer with your child or split one adult-size entrée between two children. You can also ask your server for a half portion or for half of the meal to be wrapped up to take home before it is even put on the table. Keep in mind that many restaurant serving sizes are larger than two portions—some plates might even contain four or more portions of food! Even if you eat only half, you will still consume double the amount of a healthy serving size.
- Watch the salt. Fast food, in particular, tends to be loaded with sodium. Don't add insult to injury by adding more salt.
- Save calories by ordering water or sugar-free sodas. Calories from sugary soft drinks add up fast.

Reroute Your Plate

Although it may seem like the nutritional odds are stacked against you at restaurants, you *can* take control. The solution isn't to stop eating out but to use the traffic light system to help you and your family make better food choices.

Last year I worked with 16-year-old Melissa, who was frustrated because she initially wasn't losing weight on her game plan. When we discussed her day-to-day food choices, Melissa admitted that she and her friends frequently went out to eat, but

TRAFFIC TIP

Have It Your Way!

When you sit down to eat at a restaurant, don't assume the menu is written in stone, and don't be shy about asking your server if small alterations can be made to entrées to make them healthier. These days, most restaurants are happy to oblige such requests. Here are a few examples of questions you can ask.

- Do you have a low-calorie menu?

- Can you hold the butter and oil when cooking?

- Can I have sauce, gravy, or dressing on the side?

- May I have a salad or steamed vegetable on the side instead of fries?

- Will you substitute baked or boiled potatoes for the fries?

- Can I have the chicken baked or grilled instead of fried?

- Does the ktichen trim visible fat from poultry or meat?

- Will the chef accommodate special requests?

she never knew where they'd be going in advance. Consequently, Melissa had a hard time planning and ended up eating whatever seemed good to her at the moment.

I was curious. "Do you usually go to the same few places?" I asked. She said that they typically went to a diner, a pizza place, a sushi restaurant, or a Mexican restaurant.

That was all I needed to know. Together, Melissa and I mapped out Green Light meals at each of those restaurants. That way, she always had several menu selections from which she could choose, no matter where her friends decided they wanted to go. Instead of panicking or worrying about going off her game plan, Melissa learned which foods she could safely enjoy. By planning ahead, Melissa eventually met her goal of losing 15 pounds.

For kids and teens, fast food is always a challenge. Nutritionally speaking, the problem with fast food is that it's a source of empty calories. Fast food doesn't deliver many nutrients and, in fact, typically offers little more than a combination of sugar, fat, and salt, which only stimulates us to eat more. With fast food, it's easy to consume hundreds of calories without feeling full.

The other major problem with fast food is that, as you probably know, it's very popular with kids and teens. It's cheap, convenient, and available around the clock. There are probably several fast-food restaurants near your home where kids hang out after school or on the weekends.

Matthew, an 8-year-old patient of mine, loved to eat fast food. His favorite place was Burger King, where he would order:

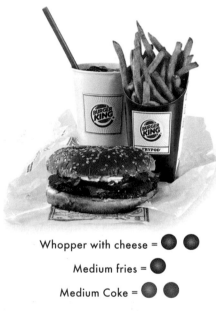

Whopper with cheese = ⚫ ⚫
Medium fries = ⚫
Medium Coke = ⚫ ⚫

Matthew was eating 1,540 calories and 71 grams of fat with each meal! When he started my program, Matthew was worried that he could never go to Burger King again. I told him that everything was okay in moderation. We decided to come up with an acceptable Burger King meal, and I explained to him that he would have to use at least one **Red Light** food when he ate there. His game plan called for four **Green Light** foods for dinner.

Below is what we decided on for his new meal.

By replacing his old meal with this lower-calorie version, Matthew could eat at Burger King once a week and still lose weight. He was so happy he was allowed to eat the food he loved that he stuck to his plan and continued to lose weight.

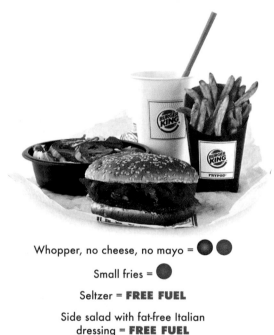

Whopper, no cheese, no mayo = ⚫ ⚫
Small fries = ⚫
Seltzer = **FREE FUEL**
Side salad with fat-free Italian dressing = **FREE FUEL**

Practically any menu item from a fast-food restaurant can be rated according to its color value—consult the Appendix for listings from many popular chains. Below you'll find more examples of restaurant food makeovers, like the ones that worked for Matthew and Melissa.

FROM RED LIGHT TO GREEN LIGHT
IN RESTAURANTS

Out to Breakfast		
STOP! ●	SLOW! ●	GO! ●
Waffle	French toast	Pancake (4 in. diameter)
Chocolate chip pancakes	Regular pancakes with syrup	Regular pancake with sugar-free syrup
Omelet with cheese	Egg white omelet with cheese	Egg white omelet with veggies, no cheese
Sausage	Bacon	Canadian bacon or turkey bacon
Hash browns/french fries	Home fries	Grits
Out to Lunch		
●	●	●
Grilled cheese sandwich	2 slices of white bread toasted (without butter or oil) with 1 slice of American cheese	Open-faced—1 slice of whole wheat bread toasted (without butter or oil) with 1 slice of American cheese
1 slice Sicilian pizza	1 small slice regular pizza	1 slice cheeseless vegetable pizza
Cheeseburger	Hamburger	French dip sandwich (take out some of the meat)
Out to Dinner—Italian		
●	●	●
Chicken parmigiana	Chicken breast (unbreaded, baked) with marinara sauce and a small amount of mozzarella cheese on top	Chicken breast, baked, with marinara sauce
Veal marsala	Veal piccata	Veal chop
Veal parmigiana	Veal scaloppine	Eggplant parmigiana (no cheese)
Penne à la vodka	Veal loin	Pasta with marinara sauce
Spaghetti carbonara	Cheese gnocchi	Potato gnocchi
Pasta primavera with cream sauce	Pasta with garlic and oil	Pasta primavera with marinara sauce

Out to Dinner—Chinese		
●	●	●
Orange chicken	Kung pao, any type	Chow mein
Orange beef	Pepper steak	Vegetables with beef, steamed
General Tso's Chicken	Moo Goo Gai Pan	Vegetables with chicken, steamed
Sweet and sour chicken, shrimp, beef, or pork	Lo mein, any type	Vegetables with shrimp or tofu, steamed
Fried rice	White rice, steamed	Brown rice, steamed
Out to Dinner—Mexican		
●	●	●
Beef tostada	Quesadilla (½)	Tamale (½)
Chuleta	Burrito, any type, large (½); fajita, chicken; or tostada, chicken (½)	Taquito, beef; beef and cheese; chicken; or chicken and cheese
Out for Fast Food		
●	●	●
Chicken Sandwich, TenderCrisp—Burger King	Salad, TenderGrill Chicken, without dressing—Burger King	Salad, Chicken Caesar, no dressing or croutons—Burger King
Chicken breast, extra crispy—KFC	Chicken wing, extra crispy—KFC	Chicken breast (no skin)—KFC
McChicken—McDonald's	Chicken McGrill without mayo—McDonald's	
Sub (6 in.), Italian, or steak and cheese—Subway	Mini sub, ham, roast beef, or turkey—Subway	Salad, chicken or ham— no dressing—Subway
Chicken Sandwich Fillet— Wendy's	Hamburger, Junior—Wendy's	Salad, Mandarin Chicken, no noodles or almonds—Wendy's

CAUTION ▸ STEER CLEAR OF THESE SALADS

Here are several examples of salads that are typically loaded with fat and calories. These are major roadblocks to weight loss!

● *Taco salad.* The beef, cheese, and sour cream make this salad a calorie nightmare—and that's before you add the large, deep-fried taco shell. If you must order one, skip the beef in favor of grilled chicken and ask for a small amount of heart-healthy guacamole and lots of salsa in place of cheese and sour cream. And don't even think about eating that taco shell!

● *Creamy salads.* These include pasta salad, potato salad, tuna salad, chicken salad, shrimp salad—any salad made with mayonnaise or sour cream. If you prepare such salads at home, opt for fat-free or low-fat mayonnaise and use it sparingly.

● *Caesar salad.* Here's a salad everyone thinks is healthy. But it is horrendous! The dressing, the cheese, and the croutons all add up to a nutritional disaster. Pass on the cheese and croutons. If possible, use a fat-free Caesar dressing or ask for another dressing, like fat-free balsamic dressing. If that is not an option, ask for the dressing on the side and use sparingly. Or make a healthy version at home using the recipe on page 142.

● *Cobb salad.* This popular salad is made with blue cheese, eggs, and bacon—a fat and cholesterol disaster! Avoid the restaurant version and make a healthy one at home with egg whites and 97 percent fat-free turkey bacon.

● *Chef salad.* This consists of about 5 ounces of roast beef, hard cheese, ham, hard-boiled egg—almost 400 calories of animal protein. A better alternative is to order a grilled chicken salad, with dressing on the side. Show your kids how to get the taste of the dressing by dipping their forks into dressing, then spearing the salad, instead of slathering their salad in dressing.

Salad Slipups

You'll find salads on the menu at almost any restaurant. But I think some should come with a warning label that reads: "Beware of excess levels of calories, fat, and sodium." Many people consider salads a healthy choice among traditional food options, but salads can do more damage to the diet than a thoughtfully chosen entrée that includes lean protein and lots of veggies.

Case in point: the Garretts, a family of three who all suffered from obesity. Nine-year-old son Todd already weighed 215 pounds. Initially, Todd was so heavy that he couldn't bend over to tie his shoes. The Garretts were all trying to lose weight, so when they went out to eat, they often ordered salads. They were puzzled and frustrated when they weren't shedding pounds.

I sat down with the Garretts and asked about the salads they ordered. After hearing their descriptions, I realized that most of those salads probably contained about 1,000 calories! No wonder they weren't losing weight. I taught them about the traffic light system and showed them how to color code each component of their salads. In turn, they adjusted the salads they ordered at restaurants. Soon everyone started losing weight. Within months, Todd could tie his shoes and run 2 miles without a problem.

Navigating a Buffet

Eating at a buffet is lots of fun, especially for kids. Children get very excited about all of the different options. How can you help your child navigate a buffet without going overboard? Here are 10 simple guidelines to help your children eat at a buffet and stick with their game plans.

1. **Don't let your child sit or stand around the buffet.** Help your child make his plate and then have him sit down at the table. Looking at the food will only make your child want to eat more.

2. **Look before you serve.** Walk around the buffet with your child and decide what she will eat before you fill the plate. Figure out which foods she likes most and stick to those. Don't put unnecessary foods on the plate.

3. **Choose a small plate,** such as a dessert or salad plate, so there is less room to load up on calories. Large plates create opportunities to pile on food.

4. **Start the buffet meal with a plate of salad** and fresh vegetables to curb hunger. Once your child is finished with the salad, then make your way to the buffet to pick main course options.

5. **Fill half your child's plate with healthy choices,** like grilled vegetables or fruit. This limits the room for fattening fare.

6. **If your kids want to use a Red Light, have them choose one unhealthy dish.** If you know your kids want to have an unhealthy dessert, make sure the rest of their meal is healthy. Don't take little bits of many different unhealthy dishes, because the calories add up quickly!

7. **Try to avoid crispy, crunchy, and creamy foods.** These foods tend to have lots of fat.

8. **Buffet foods often contain lots of sauce.** When you spoon food onto your child's plate, try to take as little sauce as possible. When possible, pick food from the top of the pan as opposed to

the bottom. Food at the bottom of the pan has been sitting in the most butter, oil, or sauce and has likely soaked up much of it.

9. **Encourage your child to eat slowly.** Don't let him shovel his food into his mouth. Teach him to focus on his food to fully enjoy the flavor.

10. **Stick with water or seltzer for drinks.** Avoid Shirley Temples and regular soda because they contain so much sugar.

Talk to Your Kids about Food Advertising

Kids today are bombarded by advertising messages and images for junk food and fast food everywhere they turn. In fact, kids see one food commercial every 5 minutes during Saturday-morning cartoons, most of them for foods high in fat, sugar, and calories.

Older kids with cell phones are even more exposed to food advertising. When they buy candy or chips, they get offers for text-based messages, free music downloads, ring tones, and whimsical wallpaper for their phone screens. They're usually routed to a Web site where they're hit with even more junk-food advertising. And the messages they get on their phones? Ads, contests, e-cards, fun phrases to forward to friends, and invitations to return to the site for more so-called freebies.

Help your kids understand this barrage of information by talking to them about food advertising. Here are some examples of questions you can ask to get the conversation started.

"Why do you think the advertiser put a commercial on this particular program?"

This gets to the heart of an important media literacy concept: All messages are designed for a particular audience.

"Why do you think advertisers use slogans or catchy music?"

You may even ask your kids to recall other songs or slogans they remember from ads. Many of us can remember a particular phrase or jingle that we heard 10 or 20 years ago.

"What is appealing in this commercial? Is it the way the food looks or the happy family seen eating the food?"

Explain tricks that advertisers use in commercials, like applying Vaseline to make hamburgers look juicy or adding chemicals to bowls of cereal to make sure the cereal doesn't get soggy. Gross! Also, explain the true purpose behind promotions, downloads, and links from games, Web sites, and cell phones. Kids need to know that no matter how clever the gimmick or game, they're all a means of selling a product.

"What might the advertiser be leaving out of the commercial and why?"

Most food ads do not communicate nutritional values. Encourage your kids to look elsewhere, such as the Internet, for the missing information.

"Does it make a difference to you that a celebrity was in that commercial?"

Teach your children about the popular techniques advertisers use, such as testimonials from celebrities—or everyday people. This will help your kids understand how they're being influenced.

Here's another idea: Consider muting the sound during commercials and asking your kids to provide dialogue. Ask, "What are they saying?" and "What music is playing?" You can also ask your kids to find subtle sponsorships and product placement in the games they play and Web sites they visit. This is a fun way to help them become more aware of popular techniques.

Think of eating out in the context of your child's game plan. If your children want to order something special, they can cut back on other meals that day. Moderation is always key, but planning ahead can help everyone enjoy dining out without sacrificing good nutrition or weight-loss goals.

10
● ● ●

FROM STOP TO GO: EXERCISE!

It seems like kids are always in the mood to play and be active, as many exhausted moms and dads can attest. As a parent, you can take advantage of these natural tendencies—and in doing so, help lay the foundation for a healthy adult life. Kids who exercise regularly are stronger and healthier than those who don't, and have a lower risk of developing diabetes, heart or circulatory diseases, and other illnesses later in life. Physically active kids even perform better in school.

Exercise burns calories, and an exercise program is essential for weight management or loss. Weight loss boils down to simple mathematics: Expend more calories than you eat. In other words, eat less and move more. The more regular and consistent a child's activity level, the more calories she will burn.

Exercise also boosts metabolism (remember, metabolism is like a furnace that burns calories all day long!) and enhances muscle mass. The more muscle someone has, the more calories he will burn, and the more fat he will lose. And what is the only way to get more muscle? Through exercise!

If your children are not natural-born athletes or don't enjoy exercising, you may have to get a little creative when it comes to physical activity. The good news is, there are plenty of activities they can choose from that don't feel like exercise at all but will provide the same health benefits. And best of all, they're fun! Your parental game plan: Find activities that match your children's interests so that they get excited about moving.

Here's an example: At 12, Meghan was big for her age, loved sugary snacks, and had trouble buttoning her clothing—all of which worried her mother. After they came to see me and Meghan started following her game plan, she lost 5 pounds! She was getting closer to her goal every day.

But it was time to start incorporating more physical activity into her plan. Like a lot of children (and adults), Meghan had tried many different exercise regimens. She hated the treadmill and refused to ride a bike. She loved to dance and took two dance classes a week, but she admitted that she spent a large amount of that time watching the instructor and waiting for her turn to practice the routine.

I decided to base her exercise routine on dancing, and together we determined that tap dancing would be the best fit for her. Not only is tap dancing a vigorous form of exercise that would get her heart rate up, but Meghan was excited to try it. These days Meghan is tapping to her heart's content. Every day she comes home from school, puts on her tap shoes, turns on her favorite music, and dances around in the basement for almost an hour. She loves it, and her weight loss has accelerated considerably. In fact, she's lost another 6 pounds!

Children like Meghan who participate in dancing, skating, team sports, gymnastics, or any activity are more likely to stay fit and maintain an active lifestyle that will carry into their adult lives. Consider enrolling your kids in an organized sport such as swimming, soccer, or basketball—but make sure it's something they will enjoy and *want* to do. If organized activities don't work for your child or your family, there are many other ways to incorporate exercise into your children's lives, and we'll look at several options in this chapter.

How Much Exercise Do Kids Really Need?

The American Academy of Pediatrics recommends that children get 60 minutes of vigorous exercise most days of the week. While this may seem like a lot, those 60 minutes don't have to be consecutive. A 20-minute bike ride to school, plus a 10-minute game of tag at recess, plus 30 minutes of after-school skateboarding adds up to 60 minutes of exercise! Don't count your child's PE class toward exercise time, however. Studies show children get an average of only 3 minutes of vigorous exercise in an average PE class.

Let's take a closer look at children's fitness needs based on age.

4- to 5-Year-Olds

Gently help younger kids appreciate exercise and develop their motor skills by leading them through sequences of basic motions. Start on two legs, with running or jumping. Then add in balancing skills, with hopping, skipping, dancing, or even somersaulting. Once kids can move their bodies with confidence, they'll be ready to try activities with other kids, like swimming classes or even neighborhood games of tag, treasure hunts, obstacle courses, or T-ball. Incorporate toys into this active play, too. Simple items like jump ropes, hula hoops, Frisbees, and balls are easy to play with anywhere. Once kids have strong motor skills, more advanced toys like pogo sticks, roller or ice skates, bikes, and swing sets with rings, ropes, and pullup bars will help develop kids' muscles and aerobic capacity.

6- to 12-Year-Olds

Kids in this age group need to build strength, coordination, and confidence. Take as many opportunities as possible to encourage active exercise and make sure your child is involved in a variety of activities, sports, and games that he or she enjoys. If your child doesn't care for organized team sports, try other challenging activities such as martial arts, fencing, golf, bicycling, skateboarding, or tennis. Encourage your kids to try a range of exercise options so that they can choose the ones they find to be the most fun. Remember that fitness should be fun at any age! Kids who enjoy sports and exercise tend to stay active throughout their lives.

Teenagers

Playing sports provides a great outlet for excess energy and helps teenagers develop social skills and build confidence outside of the classroom. Team sports, in particular, have been shown to promote personal development and healthy lifestyles.

For example, a Centers for Disease Control and Prevention (CDC) study found that high school students who take part in team sports and who are also physically active outside school may be at reduced risk for engaging in risky sexual behavior and for using drugs or cigarettes.[1] In addition, the students involved in sports had a higher chance of graduating from high school and college. These are worthwhile benefits, but I always remind parents that sports are meant to be *fun,* as well! If there is a sport your teen really enjoys and wants to take part in, encourage her to try out.

If your teen just isn't interested in team sports or feels too self-conscious to participate, there are plenty of other options for exercise that are "cool" and acceptable. Running, inline skating, tennis, cross-country skiing, hiking, rock climbing, mountain biking, yoga, Pilates, and various kinds of fitness classes are all great ways to get moving and burn calories. Unlike team sports, these are activities that they can continue to enjoy long after their high school years are over.

Some teens are interested in exercising with

weights. Weight training is something any teen can do—once kids hit puberty, their bodies begin making the hormones necessary to help build muscle in response to weight training. Having strong muscles means improved balance and coordination. It also means your teen will be less likely to get hurt if he or she plays sports. Most fitness experts recommend that teens train with light weights, since growing bones are more prone to injury. Using very heavy weights increases the chances of fracturing the growth plates at the ends of the bones. Before your child starts strength training or any other strenuous activity, however, it's a good idea to talk to your pediatrician.

Keep in mind that the right time to begin an exercise program varies according to each child and should not be based solely on age. Even though all children age the same chronologically, their physiological and motor skill development can vary a great deal. Just because your child's best friend can ride a bike without training wheels at age 6 doesn't mean that your 6-year-old should be able to do the same. Children develop skills at different ages. It's important not to compare one child to another.

Keep an Activity Diary

Parents often complain that their kids spend too much time gazing at whatever happens to be on television, playing video games, or chatting with their friends online. But most parents are unaware of how much time is actually spent engaged in these activities—which is why I recommend tracking your children's free time with an activity chart for 1 week. It will give you an accurate gauge of how your children are spending their time. Use it to monitor sedentary activities like television and computer time as well as to track your child's daily exercise.

One of my patients, 9-year-old Kimberly, loved watching TV and refused to exercise. Her parents used an activity diary to track how Kimberly was spending her free time and were shocked to discover that she was watching *4 or more* hours of television a day. No matter what her parents or I said, no matter how much we pleaded, Kimberly simply would not exercise. Finally, I told her parents to stop pressuring her. We all made a deal. We wouldn't force her to exercise as long as she agreed to limit her TV, computer, and video game time to 2 hours a day. Kimberly was thrilled and readily agreed.

I rationalized that although this wasn't ideal, anything she did would burn more calories than watching television. Her parents anxiously monitored her free time and one day discovered that she was outside playing on her swing set, climbing the rock wall, and using the monkey bars. Another day, they observed her jumping rope. Soon she was playing tag with her friends, riding her bike, and staging dance shows. Kimberly slowly began to lose weight. Simply limiting her TV and computer time forced her to pick more active hobbies.

I've included a sample activity diary below. You can write in the book, make a photocopy of this page, or re-create the chart on a large poster board and place it somewhere in your house. Keep track of your children's activities for 7 days. Then sit down and analyze the diary together. If you find that your kids aren't getting at least 60 minutes of activity a day, talk to them about activities they might like to take part in or teams they might want to join. Schedule exercise into your family's week as a set routine and make it a priority. Instead of just saying to your kids, "We should exercise four times this week," tell them, "We are exercising Mondays at 5:00 p.m. and Saturdays at 11:00 a.m.," and so forth. Kids are more likely to follow a plan with structure. As parents, it is our job to organize the family schedule and set appropriate limits to guide our children and keep them healthy.

ACTIVITY DIARY

	LENGTH OF TIME (EXACT NUMBER OF MINUTES)	TYPE OF ACTIVITY
Active exercise (face red, sweating, increased heart rate)		
Low-key activity (e.g., walks)		
Activities of daily living (e.g., gardening, chores)		
Television		
Computer (not school related)		
Computer (school related)		
Video games		

It's Your Move

My husband and I have always tried to set a positive example for our kids when it comes to exercise. We invite them to go on little runs with us, and they love to hike. One of their favorite games is "personal trainers." Zachary, my 7-year-old, pretends he is a personal trainer with his little sister, Danielle, and shows her how to lift toy dumbbells. They both think exercise is fun and that it's a game.

Whether we're intentionally teaching them or not, our children pick up many of their habits—healthy and otherwise—from watching Mom and Dad. So make sure they see you participating in physical activity in a positive way. Even when they are very young, simply riding alongside you in a jog stroller or bicycle trailer will help them to grow up with a healthy, positive outlook on fitness. And on those days when you're dreading a trip to the gym (we all have those days!), try not to let your kids hear you complain. You don't want them to grow up thinking that exercise is a chore.

Once they're old enough to join in, it's important to make exercise a family affair. With a little creative thinking, you can turn workouts into a lot of fun.

Here are some ideas to get your kids up and moving.

Go for a Ride

Try bike riding as a family. Or encourage your children to go bicycling with friends. A leisurely bike ride for 30 minutes can burn as many as 135 calories; fast bike riding can burn as many as 297 calories. This is a perfect way for your child to get a daily dose of cardiovascular exercise and have fun with friends or family at the same time.

Walk It Off

If you find it tough to get your little screen bean moving, become her fitness partner: Walk to the playground after dinner or take the family for a hike at a local park on the weekends. Walking at 2 mph for 30 minutes can burn as many as 95 calories, 3 mph 148 calories, and 4 mph 176 calories! Walking also boosts heart rate, strengthens bones and muscles, and improves stamina and fitness. Your child can burn more calories by increasing the intensity of the workout. Try walking up and down hills to increase intensity. Pedometers are great tools, because kids love to track their steps. Teach them how to use a clip-on walking meter and have them keep a progress chart. Start with 5,000 steps a day, then progress to 10,000. Eventually, he or she may aim for 20,000 steps daily.

Get Fido Involved

Give your child the chore of walking the dog and voilà—instant movement! Dogs love to run around outside. So don't even mention exercise. Just tell your kids that the dog needs to go out and suggest they take him for a walk, play chase, or even play fetch. Start by going around the block every time the dog needs to go outside. Gradually move up to longer walks. Once your pet gets used to the workout, you'll find him barking at the door, motivating your child to take him again.

Explore Exergaming

Many children find exergaming (the use of physically interactive video games) more fun than traditional forms of exercise. Examples of exergames include Wii Sports and Wii Fit. If kids use Wii Fit, for example, they progress through a series of activities that include simple yoga positions, jogging, hula hoop-ing, and ski jumping. Wii Sports games such as tennis and boxing require physical activity on the part of the gamer, making them more aerobic—and ideal for improving fitness.

I know that many parents are skeptical about the use of video games for exercise, but I believe exergaming can be a wonderful alternative to traditional exercise for many children. I see kids every day who are too embarrassed to join organized sports because they have been teased by classmates for being overweight, or whose weight prevents them from being able to be competitive with other kids. For these kids, exergaming can help them lose weight and build confidence. And on a rainy weekend afternoon, it can be an enjoyable family activity!

Dance Like the Stars

Don't underestimate the calorie burn of dancing around the house. Thirty minutes of aerobic dancing can burn as many as 202 calories and is a lot of fun. There are some excellent dance exercise DVDs you can do at home with your kids. Even if you don't have an instructional DVD, you can always turn on some music and have an impromptu dance party! A game called Dance Dance Revolution also makes a great workout—my patients love it.

Lap It Up

Swimming is a full-body workout. Swimming laps for just 20 minutes a day builds endurance and strengthens muscles. Light to moderate swimming for 30 minutes can burn from 214 to 250 calories. Swimming is good for the heart and lungs and helps to increase flexibility. Plus it's a low-impact sport, making it perfect for people rehabilitating from injuries. And kids love the water! It certainly adds a dimension of fun that can't be found in a workout on dry land. Try playing water volleyball, water polo, underwater tag, or basketball, or have swimming races.

Start Climbing

Even if you don't have a stairclimber in the house, kids can still get a stair-climbing workout by walking up and down the stairs in the house. I have a patient, Ricky, who preferred to exercise at home. Home exercise equipment wasn't within the limits of his family's budget, so Ricky got creative. He now runs up and down his stairs 30 times in a row every day. He is proud of the fact that he "made up his own exercise program." Climbing for about 30 minutes can burn up to 200 calories. (Have kids take their shoes up to their rooms while they're at it!)

Shoot Some Hoops

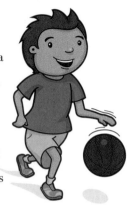

Shooting hoops or playing a group game of basketball is a fun way to get in some exercise. Don't worry about your child's skill level; it's all about moving! Shooting baskets for 30 minutes will burn up to 153 calories.

Work Out to Television

Take advantage of that time in front of the tube to exercise. Encourage your child to try marching, jogging in place, or doing jumping jacks during the program, or place some home exercise equipment in front of the TV. Some parents have their kids do jumping jacks during commercials: By the end of a 1-hour show, kids will have been jumping for 15 minutes without realizing it! Another option is to download exercise classes through online workout videos or use the free "on-demand" option on your TV. With these classes and videos, your kids can exercise anytime to hundreds of different workouts.

Red Light, Green Light, Eat Right

Try Yoga

I love to do yoga, and so do my children. They each have their own yoga mat. They'll do about 6 minutes with me; then they've had enough and will stop. My 4-year-old daughter takes a weekly yoga class for children. When the kids go into the Downward-Facing Dog position, they bark; when they do the Sun Salutation, they say, "Hi, sun!"

Children get many of the same physical benefits from yoga as adults do. Yoga strengthens muscles, improves circulation, stimulates abdominal organs, and improves breathing quality. In addition, yoga increases flexibility, coordination, energy, and bone density. Yoga can help kids develop self-awareness and improve self-esteem by allowing them to gain control over their bodies and minds at an early age. Yoga also teaches children self-discipline. During practice, children need to learn how to hold poses, breathe, and gain control of their own bodies without having external adult control. This is very empowering and motivating to children.

If you think yoga is something your son or daughter might enjoy, here are some important guidelines.

- Find the right place and teacher for your child. Talk with the instructor; are you comfortable with his or her experience? If your child is a beginner, sign her up for an introductory course. Make sure that the instructor demonstrates each pose for the children rather than simply explaining the positions.

- Use lots of positive reinforcement to help children learn and improve. Encourage doing the pose correctly, along with the breathing, but don't force perfection. Children younger than 6 years old can hold each pose for a maximum time of about 1 minute. Children 6 to 10 years old can hold each pose for a maximum time of about 1½ minutes.

- Practice in a room without mirrors. Put the emphasis on internal experience rather than outer performance.

- Allow frequent, small breaks in between and during sessions, which encourages meditation and stillness. Be sure to take breaks after strenuous exercises or poses.

- Remember, even kids need to warm up before doing vigorous yoga. Have your child march in place for 5 minutes and then jog in place for 5 minutes before beginning each yoga practice.

- Kids should not eat a full meal within 1 hour prior to class; a full tummy can be distracting and may cause nausea.

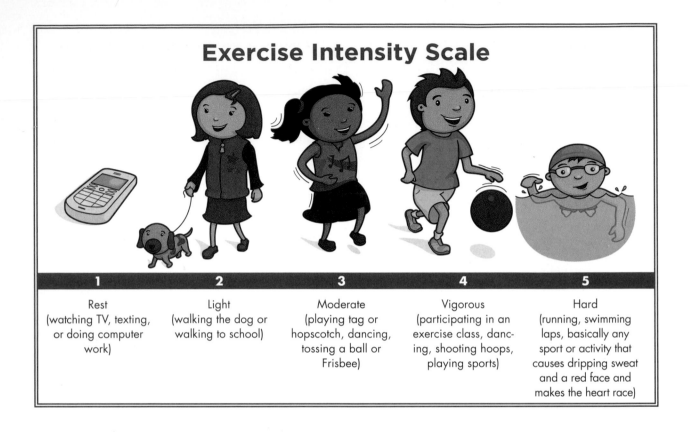

Exercise Intensity Scale

1	2	3	4	5
Rest (watching TV, texting, or doing computer work)	Light (walking the dog or walking to school)	Moderate (playing tag or hopscotch, dancing, tossing a ball or Frisbee)	Vigorous (participating in an exercise class, dancing, shooting hoops, playing sports)	Hard (running, swimming laps, basically any sport or activity that causes dripping sweat and a red face and makes the heart race)

Sneak In Exercise

There are lots of ways to burn calories through everyday activities. Here are some easy ways your child can sneak in some exercise through chores and other around-the-house tasks and the approximate number of calories they'll burn.

Get out in the garden. Weeding, mowing, and gardening for 30 minutes can burn up to 180 calories.

Hooray for housework. Thirty minutes of washing floors can burn up to 150 calories! Your house gets clean and your child gets the benefit of exercise.

Wash the car. Washing and waxing a car for 30 minutes can burn up to 154 calories and will amp up the heart rate. This is a fun family weekend activity.

Yard work. Raking leaves for 30 minutes can work the upper body and burn up to 135 calories.

Remember to have your child wear gloves to prevent blisters and show him how to bend at the knees to prevent back strain when lifting bags of leaves.

Other household tasks. Dusting can burn up to 85 calories in 30 minutes, doing laundry 73 calories, ironing 77 calories, and washing dishes 77 calories!

Exercise and Earn

If your older children are reluctant to do household or yard tasks, suggest turning these activities into a part-time job. Maybe your son or daughter can offer your neighbors services in mowing lawns (with a push mower!), shoveling snow, or raking leaves. All are great ways to get their hearts pumping, tone their upper bodies, and pad their wallets. With some portable tunes in tow, kids don't even realize they're both working and working out!

How Hard Should Kids Work Out?

Many kids may feel like they're getting good exercise when they're really not even elevating their heart rates. One way to teach your kids to gauge their exercise intensity is to use the Exercise Intensity Scale on the opposite page.

When using this scale, encourage your kids to exercise at level 4 or 5 for at least 30 minutes.

Another way to gauge physical intensity is to use the "talk test." Kids should feel winded and unable to carry on a full conversation or sing their favorite song during the peak of their activity. If they're gasping for air, their exercise intensity is too high. On the other hand, if they're able to chat with ease, it's time to kick it up a notch.

Any child, especially one who is severely overweight, should see a pediatrician or family doctor before starting an exercise program to determine a safe exercise level.

Sports Nutrition for Kids

If your children participate in sports, they need special snacks and meals to take the edge off their appetites and provide energy without leaving them too full to compete.

Water tops the list as the single most important drink for a winning performance. Kids need to drink lots of water before, during, and after a game in order to help prevent dehydration and heat exhaustion. Dehydration can occur within 30 minutes of exercise, especially in the summer months when it's hot outside. A person in a hot environment can lose up to 2 liters of fluid per hour. When possible, give your children cold water to drink, as it is absorbed by the body more easily than warm water and also helps to lower

(continued on page 208)

TRAFFIC TIP

50 Fun Ways for Everyone to Get Fit!

1. Set up backyard Olympics with activities like relay races or long jump contests.

2. Put together a simple home gym by using canned foods or books for weights.

3. Jump during TV commercials.

4. Walk around while talking on a cell phone.

5. Sign up for exercise classes or exercise to DVDs.

6. Go skateboarding.

7. Try horseback riding.

8. Play Ping-Pong.

9. Play "marching band" throughout the house.

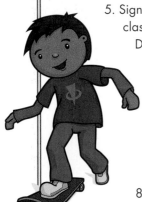

10. Go sledding.

11. Build a snowman.

12. Shovel snow.

13. Play fetch with your dog outdoors.

14. Walk in the snow or try snowshoeing.

15. Go cross-country skiing.

16. Ice-skate with friends.

17. Go inline skating or roller-skating.

18. Rock climb at a special rock-climbing gym.

19. Go on nature walks and make a game out of collecting leaves, flowers, pinecones, and so forth.

20. Make a race out of anything: Who can clean their room the fastest? Who can get dressed the fastest? Who can run to the car the fastest?

21. Blow bubbles and chase them.

22. Play hide-and-seek.

23. Set up an indoor obstacle course with chairs and pillows. Let your kids crawl and climb, stopping at activity stations for jumping jacks and pushups.

24. Play tag.

25. Use a hula hoop.

26. Take your kids to a playground.

27. Take walks in botanical gardens and nature preserves.

28. Toss a Frisbee.

29. Have your children look for rocks and twigs in the yard. Make a race out of who can find 10 items the fastest.

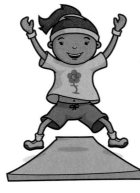

30. Play hopscotch.

31. Walk around the zoo, museum, or amusement park.

32. Try kayaking or canoeing.

33. Have a water balloon fight.

34. Have a pillow fight.

35. Sign up as a family for a charity walk or run.

36. Play miniature golf.

37. Go bowling.

38. Make a game of carrying items up and down the stairs (one person at a time).

39. Get a family membership at a local gym or health club.

40. Play tug-of-war.

41. Climb monkey bars.

42. Play Twister or Hullabaloo.

43. Challenge your child to a bicycle race; they ride and you run.

44. Play follow the leader with hopping and balancing.

45. Park far away and make a game out of reaching your destination by jogging, skipping, and tiptoeing.

46. If your destination is close by, walk (don't drive). Make sure it's safe to do so.

47. Try kickboxing (a class or video).

48. Play tennis, handball, or racquetball.

49. Use a treadmill, elliptical trainer, or stationary bike.

50. Learn to use "exercise toys," such as stability balls, medicine balls, or Bosu balls.

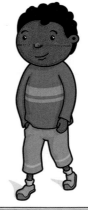

body temperature. Children older than 6 who are competing in sports should drink:

- 64 to 80 ounces of water daily
- 8 ounces of water 1 to 2 hours before exercising, and about 8 more ounces 15 minutes before
- 4 to 8 ounces of water every 15 to 20 minutes while exercising or while playing in a sports game
- 16 ounces after the game

I'm frequently asked whether kids should drink sports drinks. Sports drinks are beneficial only for children participating in intense exercise that lasts more than 90 minutes. Exercising for this length of time depletes the body of electrolytes, which are minerals that regulate where and how fluids are distributed in the body. Sports drinks contain electrolytes and are a good option for replenishing these minerals after prolonged exercise. Water, however, is just as effective at restoring the fluids lost during light or moderate exercise and keeping electrolytes in balance. In general, sports drinks provide extra sugar and calories that are not needed by children. In fact, a child who drinks a 20-ounce sports drink every day for a year can gain about 13 extra pounds!

As for food and snacks, kids should eat complex carbohydrates 1 to 4 hours before sports games. This is because carbohydrates are broken down quickly by the body and give glucose to the muscles. Some examples of complex carbohydrates are oatmeal, pasta, rice, low-sugar cereal, and whole grain bread. It is important to eat the right foods after playing sports to help muscles recover and replace the glycogen energy stores. Simple carbohydrates like a banana, granola bar, or whole grain crackers should be eaten right after exercising, followed by some protein such as a tablespoon of peanut butter, a hard-boiled egg, nuts, or turkey within a couple of hours. Eating a small amount of protein after moderate exercise helps to rebuild and repair muscle tissue that is broken down during physical activity.

Should your children eat more calories if they are actively involved in sports or other physical activities? *Unless your kids are intensively exercising for 90 or more minutes at a time, no extra calories are needed.* The quarterback of the high school football team, who practices strenuously for hours and hours each day, needs to make sure he consumes additional calories; however, most kids do not require an increased calorie intake. Just try to make sure your child eats the right foods and drinks plenty of water before and after exercise. And don't forget to count these foods as part of their color allotments!

Your child doesn't have to be an athlete to lose weight and get in shape. Any activity can be turned into vigorous exercise. Just get your kids moving! As long as your children keep active, they can enjoy a lifetime of fitness.

11

● ● ●

WINNING THE GAME: A PLAYBOOK FOR LIFE

If you've ever been on a diet, you know that the biggest challenge is not losing weight but keeping it off. Kids don't face quite the same struggle, since their set point (see page xiv) hasn't kicked in yet. Nonetheless, they do have their challenges—from attending birthday parties to going out for fast food with friends.

The best way for your children to stay at a healthy weight is to continue to choose healthy foods and follow their game plans every day. And weight loss is most likely to be successful when kids keep active.

Staying at a Healthy Weight

Remember, when you selected a game plan for your child, his or her BMI was a determining factor. The range for a healthy weight is a BMI in less than the 85th percentile. If your kids have been successful on their game plans, meaning their BMIs are in the healthy weight range, then it's time to gradually switch over to the *Red Light, Green Light, Eat Right* maintenance game plan, in which you gradually increase your child's colors. Here's an overview of how it works.

- The weight at which a child starts maintenance is his or her "goal weight."
- During week 1 of the maintenance plan, you add two **Greens** to your children's daily plan. You can add them to the snack or to the meal at which your child would most prefer to eat

a little more or have a little more freedom.

- Weigh your child once a week, at the end of the week. If his or her weight is within 2 pounds of goal, continue with the maintenance plan.
- If your child's weight is up more than 2 pounds from the goal weight, **subtract one Green** from your child's daily plan.
- If your child's weight is down more than 2 pounds from the goal, **add two Greens** to your child's daily plan.
- Do not make any changes if weight stays within 2 pounds of the goal, since it's normal for weight to fluctuate.
- Each week, your child should continue to enjoy pit stops. That means eating two **Red Light** foods!
- Your child must continue to eat a fruit or vegetable (**Free Fuel**) with each meal and snack.

Nutrition Needs during Growth Spurts

When those new pants you bought your son at the beginning of the school year are too short by Christmas, you know he's experiencing a growth spurt! Every child grows at his or her own pace. Look at your child's class picture and you'll see kids of the same age in all shapes and sizes. Some kids look tiny next to their peers, while others literally tower above their classmates. Your child's friends may look like they weigh less than your child because they have a different body type. Big, small, tall, short—there is a wide range of healthy shapes and sizes among children.

Once children reach a healthy weight, they'll actually need to gain some weight to keep up with growth spurts. As a child grows, goal weight will increase. In general, for every inch a girl grows, she should gain 5 pounds to keep her BMI the same. For every inch a boy grows, he should gain 7 pounds to maintain his BMI.

Each month, measure your child's height and adjust his or her goal weight accordingly. For example, if your daughter grows ½ inch, her goal weight should increase by 2½ pounds (or half of 5 pounds). If your son grows ½ inch, his goal weight should increase by 3½ pounds (or half of 7 pounds).

Some children are so happy with their weight loss that they might be reluctant to add more food into their game plans. Kimberly, age 8, is a good example. She had been overweight almost since birth. She desperately wanted to be in shape like her friends, and she followed her game plan with gusto. As a result of her dedication, she brought her BMI down from an unhealthy 97 percent to a healthy 80 percent in 6 months. She was thrilled that she had met her goal, but she was nervous about adding more foods into

More Ways to Stay in Shape

● **EAT FREE FUEL IN THE FORM OF FRUITS AND VEGGIES EVERY DAY.** When your family eats more fruits and vegetables while cutting back on high-fat, high-sugar foods, everyone will slim down. That's the conclusion of a study published in the journal *Obesity Research*.[1] Parents who introduced more fruits and veggies into their family meals, while decreasing fat and sugar, lost weight, and so did their kids.

● **DON'T SKIP MEALS, ESPECIALLY BREAKFAST.** Breakfast kick-starts the metabolism, burning calories from the get-go and providing energy throughout the day. Kids who skip breakfast often feel so hungry that they eat more later on. And people who skip breakfast tend to have higher BMIs than people who eat break-fast. When you don't eat, you slow down your metabolism. Eating regular healthy meals helps keep your metabolism up and burning more energy.

● **PAY ATTENTION TO PORTION SIZES.** If a portion is large, encourage kids to cut it in half and put half aside for later—or split it with a friend.

● **GET SUPPORT.** Encourage your children to find others who support them in losing weight and staying healthy. Support helps us feel better about ourselves, and feeling better about ourselves helps us lose weight and keep it off.

● **STAY ACTIVE!** Your children are far more likely to get and stay slim if they accept that exercise must be an everyday part of life. Have a daily family fun time—even something as simple as a family walk after dinner will get your kids up and moving instead of vegging out for the evening in front of the TV.

---

her game plan because she was afraid she would regain the weight she'd worked so hard to lose.

I spoke with Kimberly and encouraged her to gradually add foods to her game plan. I told her that a small amount of weight gain would be normal, and if that occurred, it was no reason to panic. Sure enough, when she gained 2 pounds one month, she became hysterical. I sat down with her and we looked at her growth chart. Kimberly had grown a full inch in just a few months—which meant her BMI had actually *decreased!* Once I pointed out the pattern of her height and weight gain over time, she felt better and could see that she was progressing normally. Kimberly continued to follow a maintenance game plan, gradually added in more foods, and has kept the weight off ever since.

Even kids as young as Kimberly can become overly concerned about weight gain once they have managed to lose excess pounds. Talk to your children about their feelings and explain to them that it's okay if they gain or lose a couple of pounds—that's normal. Help them understand that *health* is the priority, not weight.

Lots of factors—genetics, gender, nutrition, physical activity, health problems, environment, and hormones—influence a child's height and weight. That's why it's a good idea to involve your family doctor or pediatrician when you make changes to your child's diet. If you have any questions about your child's growth or weight, talk with your doctor. Using growth charts, your physician can help you understand the pattern of your child's height and weight gain over time and determine whether his or her development is healthy.

Going Off-Road: Slipups!

If your child goes off his game plan and gains weight, don't panic or make him feel guilty. Reassure him that slipups are normal and encourage him to forgive himself. Then, as soon as possible, get right back on the game plan. If your child consciously makes small, healthy changes, eventually they will become habits again.

Slipups can provide valuable learning experiences. Sit down with your child and take a look at behaviors that might have led to the detour. For example:

- Did she have too many sugary drinks? Look at ways to replace soft drinks, fruit juices, and sports drinks that are loaded with sugar with the less-caloric beverages mentioned throughout the book.
- Did he eat too many big portions of food at fast-food restaurants? If so, talk about ways to make healthier fast-food choices. Pick a small, single-patty burger instead of a large one, and a side salad instead of fries. And stick to regular servings—don't supersize!
- Has she been snacking on too many Red Light foods during the week? Make sure your child packs good-for-you snacks so she avoids food vending machines. Try carrot sticks, a piece of fruit, or your own homemade trail mix instead of cookies, chips, or processed foods that tend to be loaded with fat and calories.
- Did he stop riding his bicycle because it was too boring doing the same thing all the time? Suggest a new form of exercise to get him interested in moving again.

Managing these situations is a key part of maintaining weight loss. For example, when 12-year-old

Brian lost 30 pounds and reached his goal weight after following his game plan for more than a year, he thought he could go back to his old eating habits and remain healthy. For 2 weeks, Brian went off his game plan entirely, eating lots of fast food and junk food with his friends.

When Brian checked in with me, he had regained 5 pounds and was devastated. He admitted to me that his stomach "didn't feel good," most likely a result of the junky food he had been eating. I put him back on his original game plan until he dropped those 5 pounds; then I gradually switched him to his maintenance plan, slowly adding in colors until his weight was stable. When that happened, Brian was able to eat more snacks with his friends and enjoy some fast food each week, as long as he paid attention to what he ordered. He was thrilled and has kept his weight off ever since.

If your child regains weight, look at her eating and exercise habits, make adjustments, and get back on track.

Emotional Eating

We're all familiar with the urge to turn to food as a source of celebration or comfort—grown-ups do it, and kids do it, too. Sometimes we eat not because we're hungry but simply because we feel happy, sad, bored, stressed, or lonely. Everyone emotionally eats sometimes, but if this type of eating becomes habitual, it will lead to weight gain. If you feel your child has a tendency to turn to food when he is feeling heightened emotions, try the following techniques.

Pay Close Attention to Triggers

Triggers are events that may lead to emotional eating. Talk to your children about why they might be eating when they aren't hungry. Do they mindlessly snack on crackers or cereal when they feel stressed from too much homework? Do fights with friends trigger cravings for sweets like ice cream? When they have nothing to do on a Saturday and are bored, do they graze on chips? If so, they are looking for food to make them less stressed and help them feel comforted or occupied. Food, of course, doesn't really do any of those things; in the end, it can make the problem worse. Talk to your children about healthy ways to deal with emotions and boredom, like scheduling something fun to do after school or at night, reading a book, keeping a journal, exercising, or talking with a friend. Help your child see food for what it is—a way to fuel the body.

Use the Hunger and Fullness Scales

Listening to the body's signals of hunger and fullness can help minimize emotional eating. Talk to your kids about eating only when truly hungry. If they feel like munching but admit that they aren't physically hungry, it's time to do something that will take their minds off food, like play a game, call a friend, or watch a movie—any option that doesn't include food. On the other hand, if your child is truly hungry, let her eat. Even if it's not time for a regular meal or snack, pay attention to internal hunger cues. Your kids will more fully enjoy their food when they are truly hungry.

Do Not Forbid Food

One reason traditional diets fail is because they often encourage people to think of foods as "good" or "bad." There are no good or bad foods, but there *are* good and bad portions. Most diets also encourage people to avoid so-called bad foods, and that can lead to feelings of deprivation and out-of-control cravings. Don't deny your children certain foods—it will only increase their desire to eat them and to overindulge when they do. Occasional treats are an essential part of the *Red Light, Green Light, Eat Right* plan. A Red Light food like a candy bar will taste more special if it's a once-in-a-while treat instead of an everyday snack.

Deal with Depression

We like to think of childhood as a happy, carefree time, but as a doctor, I can tell you that depression is on the rise in children. I believe one reason for this is because mental health is strongly tied to physical health. Being overweight can be hard, both physically and emotionally, on a child. And when it comes to weight loss, occasional slipups can leave children feeling discouraged and disappointed. This, in turn, may lead to self-criticism, anger, or even guilt about letting friends or family down. If your child seems mad or irritable, doesn't enjoy favorite activities anymore, has trouble sleeping, withdraws socially, or complains of stomach pain or headaches for a week or longer, he or she may be depressed. If you suspect your child is depressed, talk to your pediatrician, who may refer you to a child therapist. Talking things over can help children figure out how to deal with powerful emotions.

The College Years: Beating the Freshman 15

If you're a parent of teens, I'm sure you've heard warnings about the infamous "freshman 15." But is it true that college students pack on 15 pounds during their first year at school? And if so, how can your child avoid weight gain once they leave home?

Recent studies confirm that some first-year students indeed gain weight—but it might not be the full freshman 15. Other students tend to gain weight gradually throughout their 4 years of college—which is less dramatic, but still dangerous, as it may lead to a pattern of weight gain over time. Some weight gain at college is normal. Even though our sons and daughters seem grown-up at 17 to 18 years old, they are still growing out of adolescence, and their metabolisms are shifting. But pronounced or rapid weight gain is not healthy.

College offers many temptations. Students are on their own and are free to eat and drink what they want, when they want it. The dining hall provides the opportunity for large portion sizes and dinners of french fries and ice cream, and many a late-night study session is fueled by extra-large lattes and sugary, salty snacks. In addition, unless they play sports, college students may not get as much exercise as they did in high school. Here are some easy ways for your college-bound kids to squeeze activity into their day.

- Walk or bike to class as much as possible, instead of driving or taking the campus bus.
- Take the stairs instead of elevators in class buildings and dorms.
- Participate in an intramural sport such as volleyball; this is an enjoyable way to stay active, burn calories, and make new friends.
- Find out about open pool hours and squeeze in a few laps between classes.

- Enlist a friend to go to the gym—students will be more apt to stick with a regimen if they have workout buddies. Most college campuses have gyms and exercise classes that are free to full-time students.
- Sign up for a physical education elective, like yoga, weight training, or track.
- Check out the local YMCA—many offer fitness classes at a discount to students.

When college students gain weight, they are often tempted to go on crash diets or skip meals to lose it. But these approaches don't keep weight off in the long run. I advise all my college-bound patients to continue to use the traffic light system to maintain their weight away from home. For example, 17-year-old Melanie had just reached her goal weight before leaving for college. Understandably, she was worried about keeping off the pounds while at school. Melanie had already learned about healthy nutrition, and she knew what an appropriate serving size looked like. She had all the tools she needed. I told her to just keep doing what she had been doing. Melanie was able to fix most of her meals in the dorm kitchen, so she continued to follow her game plan. She always saved her Red Light foods for weekends and late-night snacking. The program is so flexible and allows for so many foods that her friends never knew Melanie was on a weight management plan. And she didn't gain the freshman 15!

Gaining weight as a college student is not inevitable. Students may have their ups and downs, but as long as they stay on their game plans and stay physically active, they can remain at a healthy weight.

A Game Plan for Life

You and your family are now armed with the road map to a healthy life. Start looking at healthy, nutritious foods as desirable foods. Make small, gradual changes every day. Integrate new meal and snack habits and increased physical activity into your family's structure and lifestyle. And above all, enjoy the journey!

This is what I advise the parents of my patients: *You* are responsible for deciding what foods are available in your home and when. When you follow the recommendations laid out in the *Red Light, Green Light, Eat Right* program, you can avoid daily struggles over snacks and second helpings. Your whole family will benefit from these changes and will get slimmer, healthier, happier, and more energetic. The program provides lifestyle habits you can live with, so that everyone can enjoy a long life free of obesity and obesity-related diseases. For many kids struggling with weight, this program will help them to attain a level of health and fitness—not to mention happiness and confidence—that may have previously seemed out of reach. In addition to these many benefits, you'll have fun and become closer as a family. Everyone wins!

Appendix

● ● ●

The *Red Light, Green Light, Eat Right* Food Database

The following database lists the traffic light values and serving sizes for more than a thousand foods, grouped by categories such as dairy foods, proteins, starches, snacks, ethnic foods, and fast foods.

If you're trying to locate a specific food, flip to its larger category, then look for it listed alphabetically. For example, if you're looking for Cheerios, you would look under "Breakfast Foods" and then "Cereal." Specific cereals are listed alphabetically, and you'll easily find Cheerios.

The database's fast-food category is set up for easy navigation. Under this category, foods are listed alphabetically by restaurant. So if you want to learn about the color values of foods at McDonald's, turn to the Fast Food heading, and then go down the list alphabetically until you find the section for McDonald's. All of the McDonald's entries are listed alphabetically.

Every food is color coded to make it easy to identify the healthiest alternatives. This database gives you every piece of information you need to adopt the *Red Light, Green Light, Eat Right* program. In no time at all, you and your family will be planning, preparing, and enjoying a huge variety of foods while losing weight and getting healthy.

Don't forget, items with an * indicate recommended foods that are the most nutritious choices.

* Indicates most nutritious option

BREAKFAST FOODS
CEREAL

All cereals include ¼ c of fat-free milk.

Food	Amount	
All-Bran*	⅔ c	●
All-Bran with Extra Fiber	1 c	●
Alpha Bits	¾ c	●
Apple Cinnamon Squares	½ c	●
Banana Nut Crunch	¾ c	●
Basic 4*	½ c	●
Blueberry Morning	⅔ c	●
Boo Berry	¾ c	●
Bran 100%*	½ c	●
Bran Flakes*	¾ c	●
Cap'n Crunch	⅔ c	●
Cheerios, Regular and Multi-Grain*	¾ c	●
Cheerios, All Other Types Not Listed	¾ c	●
Cheerios, Apple Cinnamon	⅔ c	●
Chex, Corn	¾ c	●
Chex, Frosted Mini	⅔ c	●
Chex, Multi-Bran*	⅔ c	●
Chex, Rice or Wheat	1 c	●
Cinnamon Grahams	⅔ c	●
Cinnamon Oatmeal Squares*	¾ c	●
Cinnamon Toast Crunch	½ c	●
Cocoa Blasts	¾ c	●
Cocoa Krispies	⅔ c	●
Cocoa Pebbles	⅔ c	●
Cocoa Puffs	¾ c	●
Cookie Crisp, Any Flavor	¾ c	●
Corn Flakes, Country	¾ c	●

Food	Amount	
Corn Flakes, Regular	1 c	●
Corn Pops	¾ c	●
Count Chocula	¾ c	●
Cracklin' Oat Bran*	⅔ c	●
Cranberry Macadamia Nut*	¾ c	●
Cream of Wheat*	1 c	●
Crispix	¾ c	●
Crispy Wheats 'n Raisins*	½ c	●
Crunchberries	⅔ c	●
Crunchy Bran*	¾ c	●
Fiber One*	¾ c	●
Frankenberry	¾ c	●
French Toast Crunch	⅔ c	●
Froot Loops	⅔ c	●
Frosted Flakes	⅔ c	●
Frosted Krispies	⅔ c	●
Frosted Mini Wheats, Bite-Size*	½ c	●
Fruit & Fiber	½ c	●
Fruity Pebbles	⅔ c	●
Golden Crisp	⅔ c	●
Golden Grahams	⅔ c	●
Granola	⅓ c	●
Granola, Fruit, Low-Fat*	⅔ c	●
Granola, Low-Fat*	¼ c	●
Granola, Low-Fat, with Raisins*	¼ c	●
Grape-Nuts Flakes*	⅔ c	●
Grape-Nuts*	½ c	●
Great Grains, Crunchy Pecan*	⅔ c	●
Great Grains, Raisin, Date & Pecan*	⅔ c	●
Harmony	⅔ c	●
Honey Bunches of Oats	⅔ c	●

Honeycomb	1 c	●	Oatmeal, Plain*	¾ c	●
Honey Crunch Corn Flakes	⅔ c	●	Oatmeal, Plain, Instant*	1 packet	●
Honey Graham Ohs!	⅔ c	●	Oatmeal, Weight Control*	1 packet	●
Honey Nut Clusters*	½ c	●	Oatmeal Crisp, Almond*	½ c	●
Just Right, Fruit & Nut*	½ c	●	Oatmeal Crisp, Apple*	½ c	●
Kaboom	1 c	●	Oatmeal Crisp, Raisin*	½ c	●
Kashi Flakes*	½ c	●	Oatmeal Squares*	½ c	●
Kashi GoLean*	⅔ c	●	Optimum*	½ c	●
Kashi GoLean Crunch*	½ c	●	Optimum Slim*	½ c	●
Kashi Good Friends*	½ c	●	Oreo O's	⅔ c	●
Kashi Heart to Heart*	⅔ c	●	Peanut Butter Crunch	⅔ c	●
Kashi Honey Puffs*	¾ c	●	Puffed Wheat	2 c	●
Kashi Honey Sunshine*	¾ c	●	Puffins*	¾ c	●
Kashi Mighty Bites*	¾ c	●	Raisin Bran*	½ c	●
Kashi Nuggets*	½ c	●	Raisin Bran Crunch*	⅔ c	●
Kashi Puffs*	1¼ c	●	Raisin Nut Bran*	½ c	●
King Vitamin	1¼ c	●	Raisin Squares Mini-Wheats*	¾ c	●
Kix	1 c	●	Reese's Peanut Butter Puffs	½ c	●
Kix, Berry Berry	⅔ c	●	Rice Krispies	1 c	●
Life, Oat Cinnamon	⅔ c	●	Shredded Wheat*	½ c	●
Life, Oat	⅔ c	●	Shredded Wheat, Frosted*	½ c	●
Lucky Charms	¾ c	●	Shredded Wheat'n Bran*	⅔ c	●
Mini-Wheats, Non-Frosted*	⅔ c	●	Smacks	⅔ c	●
Natural Cereal 100%, Oats & Honey*	¼ c	●	Smart Start	½ c	●
Natural Cereal 100%, Oats, Honey & Raisins*	¼ c	●	Special K	¾ c	●
Nestle Nesquick Cereal, Chocolate	⅔ c	●	Special K, Red Berries	¾ c	●
Oat Bran Flakes, Common Sense*	⅔ c	●	Strawberry Squares Mini-Wheats*	¾ c	●
Oat Bran*	½ c	●	Sweet Puffs	¾ c	●
Oatmeal, Flavored	1 packet	●	Toasted Oatmeal, Honey Nut*	½ c	●
Oatmeal, Flavored, Lower-Sugar*	1 packet	●	Total	¾ c	●
			Total, Brown Sugar and Oat	⅔ c	●

Total, Corn	1 c	●
Total, Whole Grain*	⅔ c	●
Trix	¾ c	●
Waffle Crisp	¾ c	●
Wheat Bran Flakes*	¾ c	●
Wheaties*	¾ c	●
Wheaties Energy Crunch*	½ c	●
Wheaties, Honey Frosted	⅔ c	●
OTHER BREAKFAST FOODS		
Cinnamon Roll, Pillsbury	1	●
French Toast, Restaurant or Homemade	1	●
French Toast Sticks, Frozen	1	●
Grits	⅔ c	●
Grits, Instant, Original	1 packet	●
Muffin, Large	½	●
Muffin, Mini	1	●
Muffin Tops, Frozen, Mini	3	●
Pancake (4" diameter)	1	●
Pancake (6" diameter)	1	●
Pancake, Frozen	1	●
Pancakes, Frozen, Mini	4	●
Syrup, Low-Calorie	¼ c	●
Syrup, Regular	2 Tbsp	●
Syrup, Sugar-Free	Unlimited	Free
Waffle, Frozen, French Toast Style	1	●
Waffle, Frozen, Low-Fat	1	●
Waffle, Frozen, Nutri-Grain, Regular* or Low-Fat*	1	●
Waffle, Frozen, Regular	1	●
Waffles, Frozen, Mini	4	●
Waffles, Restaurant or Homemade	1½	●

DAIRY		
CHEESE		
American	1 slice	●
American, 2%*	2 slices	●
American, Fat-Free*	Unlimited	Free
Babybel, Mini	1	●
Blintz, Cheese	1	●●
Cottage Cheese, 1% Milkfat	⅔ c	●
Cottage Cheese, 4% Milkfat	½ c	●
Cottage Cheese, Fat-Free*	¾ c	●
Cream Cheese	2 Tbsp	●
Cream Cheese, Fat-Free	⅓ c	●
Cream Cheese, Low-Fat	3 Tbsp	●
Cream Cheese, Soy	2 Tbsp	●
Cream Cheese, Whipped	2 Tbsp	●
Feta	3 Tbsp	●
Grilled Cheese Sandwich, Restaurant	1	●●
Hard Cheese, Fat-Free (1" cubes)*	Unlimited	Free
Hard Cheese, Fat-Free, Shredded*	Unlimited	Free
Hard Cheese, Fat-Free, Sliced*	Unlimited	Free
Hard Cheese, Low-Fat or Soy (1" cubes)*	1½	●
Hard Cheese, Low-Fat or Soy, Shredded*	½ c	●
Hard Cheese, Low-Fat or Soy, Sliced*	1½	●
Hard Cheese, Regular (1" cubes)	1	●
Hard Cheese, Regular, Shredded	⅓ c	●
Hard Cheese, Regular, Sliced	1	●
Laughing Cow, Light*	3	●
Laughing Cow, Regular	2	●

Mozzarella, Fat-Free*	Unlimited	Free
Mozzarella, Fried	2 pieces	●
Mozzarella, Part-Skim*	¼ c	●
Mozzarella, Regular	¼ c	●
Parmesan, Grated	¼ c	●
Ricotta, Fat-Free*	Unlimited	Free
Ricotta, Part-Skim*	⅓ c	●
Ricotta, Whole	¼ c	●
String Cheese, Part-Skim or Regular*	1	●
MILK AND BUTTER		
Butter, Light	1 Tbsp	●
Butter, Regular	1½ Tbsp	●
Butter, Whipped, Regular	1 Tbsp	●
Buttermilk, 1% or 2%	1 c	●
Chocolate Milk, Low-Fat	⅔ c	●
Chocolate Milk, Soy	1 c	●
Chocolate Milk, Whole	1 c	●
Cream, Half-and-Half, Fat-Free	⅔ c	●
Cream, Half-and-Half, Regular	¼ c	●
Cream, Heavy	⅓ c	●
Cream, Light	⅓ c	●
Margarine, Fat-Free	Unlimited	Free
Margarine, Hard	1½ Tbsp	●
Margarine, Reduced-Calorie	1 Tbsp	●
Margarine, Soft	1½ Tbsp	●
Milk, 1% Fat	¾ c	●
Milk, 2% Fat	⅔ c	●
Milk, Fat-Free*	1 c	●
Milk, Soy, Fat-Free*	1½ c	●
Milk, Soy, Light*	1¼ c	●

Milk, Soy, Regular	1 c	●
Milk, Whole	½ c	●
YOGURT AND SOUR CREAM		
Sour Cream	⅓ c	●
Sour Cream, Fat-Free	½ c	●
Sour Cream, Light	¼ c	●
Yogurt, Danimals*	1 container	●
Yogurt, Fruit-Flavored, Fat-Free (4 oz container)*	1	●
Yogurt, Fruit-Flavored, Low-Fat (4 oz container)*	1	●
Yogurt, Fruit-Flavored, Fat-Free (6 oz container)*	1	●
Yogurt, Fruit-Flavored, Low-Fat (6 oz container)*	1	●
Yogurt, Go-Gurt*	1	●
Yogurt, Plain, Fat-Free (4 oz or 6 oz container)*	1	●
Yogurt, Plain, Low-Fat (4 oz or 6 oz container)*	1	●
Yogurt, Plain, Whole Milk (4 oz container)	1	●
Yogurt, Plain, Whole Milk (6 oz container)	1	●
Yogurt, Soy, Flavored or Plain (4 oz container)*	1	●
Yogurt, Soy, Flavored or Plain (6 oz container)*	1	●
Yogurt, Yo Crunch, Light	1 container	●
Yogurt, Yo Crunch	1 container	●
Yogurt, Yoplait Kids*	1 container	●
Yogurt, Yoplait Kids, Yogurt Drink*	1 bottle	●
Yogurt, Yoplait, Thick and Creamy	1 container	●
Yogurt, Yo Plus	1 container	●

PROTEIN		
EGGS		
Egg*	1	●
Egg Salad	½ c	●
Egg Whites*	4	●
FISH		
Cod*	3 oz	●
Fish, most types*	3 oz	●
Fish, Fried, Breaded with Flour	3 oz	●
Fish Sticks	5	●
Flounder*	3 oz	●
Gefilte Fish*	1 piece	●
Halibut*	2½ oz	●
Lox*	2 oz (~5 small slices)	●
Salmon*	2 oz	●
Shellfish*	1 c	●
Shrimp, Cooked without Oil*	6 large	●
Shrimp, Fried	3 medium	●
Shrimp Scampi	5 medium	●
Snapper*	3 oz	●
Sole*	3 oz	●
Swordfish*	2 oz	●
Tilapia*	2 oz	●
Tuna, Canned in Oil	⅔ can	●
Tuna, Canned in Water*	½ can	●
Tuna Salad	½ c	●
Tuna Steak*	2½ oz	●
MEAT, MEAT DISHES, AND LUNCH MEATS		
Bacon	3 slices	●
Bacon, Canadian-Style	2 slices	●

Beef, Ground, Regular (75%), Cooked	½ c (2 oz)	●
Beef, Ground, Regular (75%), Raw	4 oz	●
Beef, Ground, 80% Lean, Cooked	½ c (2 oz)	●
Beef, Ground, 80% Lean, Raw	4 oz	●
Beef, Ground, 85% Lean, Cooked	⅔ c (2½ oz)	●
Beef, Ground, 85% Lean, Raw	4 oz	●
Beef, Ground, 90% Lean, Cooked	¾ c (3 oz)	●
Beef, Ground, 90% Lean, Raw	4 oz	●
Beef, Ground, 93% Lean, Cooked (Extralean)*	½ c (2 oz)	●
Beef, Ground, 93% Lean, Raw (Extralean)*	2 oz	●
Beef, Ground, 95% Lean, Cooked (Extralean)*	½ c (2 oz)	●
Beef, Ground, 95% Lean, Raw (Extralean)*	3 oz	●
Beef, Ground Sirloin, Cooked	⅔ c	●
Beef, Round	3 oz	●
Beef Stew	½ c	●
Beef Stir-Fry	½ c	●
Bologna	2 slices	●
Bologna, Fat-Free	5 slices	●
Bologna, Turkey	3 slices	●
Brisket	1½ slices	●
Burger, with Roll, Medium	1	●
Cabbage, Stuffed, Meat	1	●●
Cholent, Meat	1 large serving	●●●
Chopped Liver	¼ c	●
Chorizo	4" link	●
Corned Beef	1 slice	●

Food	Serving
Filet Mignon, Trimmed of Fat	2 oz
Flank Steak, Lean, Trimmed of Fat*	3 oz (1½ slices)
Ham, Lean*	2 oz
Ham, Lunch Meat*	4 slices
Ham, Regular	3 oz (1½ slices)
Hot Dog, 97% Fat-Free (without Roll)	2
Hot Dog, 100% Fat-Free (without Roll)	2
Hot Dog, Reduced-Fat (without Roll)	1
Hot Dog, Regular (without Roll)	1
Lamb, Cooked, Lean, Fat Trimmed, Chops or Sliced	3 oz
Lamb, Cooked, Regular, Chops or Sliced	2 oz
Lamb Leg Shank	4 oz
Lamb Stew	¾ c
Meatballs, No Sauce, Large	1½
Meatballs, Turkey, No Sauce*	3
Meatloaf, Sliced (½" thick)	1 slice
Pastrami, Regular	4 slices
Pastrami, Turkey	3 slices
Pork, Lean Cuts, Trimmed, Chops or Sliced*	3 oz
Pork, Regular, Chops or Sliced	3 oz
Pork, Regular, Sliced	1½
Pork Tenderloin*	2 oz
Pot Roast	2 oz
Ribs, Barbecued	3
Ribs, Short	1
Roast Beef	2 oz
Roast Beef, Lunch Meat, Thin Sliced*	4
Salami, Hard	4 slices
Salami, Soft	3 slices

Food	Serving
Sausage, Beef or Pork, Patties or Links	1½ pieces
Sausage, Chorizo	4" link
Sausage, Italian	1½ links
Short Ribs, Trimmed of Fat	1 rib
Sirloin*	3 oz (1½ slices)
Sirloin, Ground, Cooked	⅔ c
Souvlaki	1 large skewer
Steak, Lean, Trimmed (e.g., Round, Loin)*	3 oz
Steak, Regular	2½ oz
Steak, Skirt*	3 oz
Steak, T-Bone	1 small (3 oz)
Veal Cutlet, Breaded and Fried	2 oz
Veal Loin, Lean*	2 oz
Veal Loin, Regular*	3 oz
Veal Marsala	⅔ serving
Veal Parmigiana	⅔ piece
Veal Piccata	1 slice
Veal Scaloppine	1 slice
Veal, Trimmed, Chops*	1½
Veal, Trimmed, Sliced*	1½

POULTRY AND POULTRY DISHES

Food	Serving
Chicken Biryani	½ c
Chicken Breast, BBQ, No Skin*	½ (2 oz)
Chicken Breast, Cooked, No Skin*	½ (2 oz)
Chicken Breast, Cooked, with Skin	¾ (3 oz)
Chicken Breast, Fried, with Skin	¾ (3 oz)
Chicken, Buffalo Wings	1
Chicken Cacciatore	½ c

Chicken Cordon Bleu	3 oz	●
Chicken Cutlet, Breaded, Fried	¾ (3 oz)	●
Chicken, Dark Meat, No Skin*	1½ slices	●
Chicken, Dark Meat, No Skin*	⅔ c	●
Chicken, Dark Meat, No Skin*	¼ chicken	●
Chicken Drumstick, Cooked, with Skin	1	●
Chicken Drumstick, Cooked, without Skin*	1½	●
Chicken Drumstick, Fried, with Skin	1	●
Chicken Fingers	1	●
Chicken Francese	¾ piece	●
Chicken, Ground, Cooked*	⅓ c	●
Chicken, Ground, Raw*	2 oz	●
Chicken Marsala	½ piece	●
Chicken Nuggets, Fried	3	●
Chicken Nuggets, Frozen, Baked	2	●
Chicken Nuggets, Frozen, Baked, Whole Wheat	2	●
Chicken Parmigiana, with Sauce	4 oz	●
Chicken, Roasted, with Skin	¼ chicken	●
Chicken Salad	⅓ c	●
Chicken, Sweet-and-Sour	⅔ c	●
Chicken Thigh, BBQ, with Skin	1	●
Chicken Thigh, Cooked, with Skin	1	●
Chicken Thigh, Cooked, without Skin*	1½	●
Chicken Thigh, Fried, with Skin	1	●
Chicken, White Meat, without Skin, Chopped*	½ c	●
Chicken, White Meat, without Skin, Sliced*	1	●
Chicken Wing, Cooked, with Skin	1	●
Chicken Wing, Fried, with Skin	1	●
Duck, Cooked, Skinless	⅓ duck	●

Duck, Cooked, with Skin, ¼ Duck	⅔ item	●
Stir-Fried Chicken with Vegetables, without Oil*	1 c	●
Turkey Bacon	2 slices	●
Turkey, Breast, Cooked, with Skin	2 oz	●
Turkey, Dark Meat, Skinless, Chopped*	½ c	●
Turkey, Dark Meat, Skinless, Sliced*	3 oz	●
Turkey, Dark Meat, with Skin	3 oz	●
Turkey, Ground, 93%, Cooked*	½ c (2 oz)	●
Turkey, Ground, 93%, Raw*	2 oz	●
Turkey, Ground, 99%, Cooked*	½ c (3 oz)	●
Turkey, Ground, 99%, Raw*	4 oz	●
Turkey, Ground, Regular, Cooked	⅔ c (2 oz)	●
Turkey, Ground, Regular, Raw	4 oz	●
Turkey, Ground, White Meat, Cooked*	½ c (3 oz)	●
Turkey, Ground, White Meat, Raw*	3 oz	●
Turkey, Hot Dog, Fat-Free (without Roll)	2	●
Turkey, Hot Dog, Regular (without Roll)	1	●
Turkey Meatballs, Frozen	2	●
Turkey Salami	3 slices	●
Turkey, White Meat, Skinless, Sliced*	2 oz	●
Turkey, Wing, with Skin	¾	●
VEGETARIAN PROTEIN		
Burger, Veggie, Regular, without Bun*	1	●
Cabbage, Stuffed, Vegetarian	1	●
Cholent, Vegetarian	1 large serving	● ●
Sausage, Links, Vegetarian	3	●
Sausage, Patties, Vegetarian	2	●

Tofu*	½ c	●
Tofu, Low-Fat*	⅔ c	●

STARCHES
BREAD

Bagel, Large	½	●
Bagel, Mini	1	●
Bagel, Small	1 (2 oz)	●
Banana Bread	1 slice (3 oz)	●●
Bialy	1	●
Biscuit (2½" diameter)	1	●
Biscuit (4" diameter)	½	●
Bread Crumbs, Plain or Seasoned	⅓ c	●
Breadsticks, Hard	2	●
Breadsticks, Soft, Regular or Garlic	1	●
Callah (Saffron Loaf)	1 slice	●
Challah Bread	1 slice (2 oz)	●
Challah Roll	1 (4 oz)	●●
Charoset	½ c	●
Cinnamon Raisin Bread	1 slice	●
Corn Bread	2 oz piece	●
Croissant, Plain, Medium	1	●●
Croutons, Fat-Free	½ c	●
Croutons, Regular	⅓ c	●
Dinner Roll, Egg, Wheat, or White	1 (1 oz)	●
English Muffin	1	●
English Muffin, Light*	1	●
Flagel	½	●

Focaccia	3 oz	●●
Garlic Bread, Frozen	1 slice (2 oz)	●
Garlic Bread, Homemade or Restaurant	1 small slice (2 oz)	●
Hamburger Bun, Light	1	●
Hamburger Bun, Regular	1	●
High Fiber (>3 g per slice)*	1 slice	●
Hot Dog Bun	1	●
Hot Dog Bun, Light	1	●
Italian Bread	1 slice	●
Kaiser Roll	1	●
Matzo	¾ board	●
Matzo Ball	1 medium	●
Matzo Meal	½ c	●●
Kugel, Matzo	1 small square	●●
Pita, Small*	1	●
Potato Bread	1 slice	●
Reduced-Calorie Bread, Any Type*	2 slices	●
Rye Bread, Regular*	1 slice	●
Rye Bread, Thinly Sliced*	2 slices	●
Stuffing, Bread, from Mix	½ c	●
Tortilla, Corn (6" diameter)	2	●
Tortilla, Wheat (6" diameter)	1	●
Tortilla, Wheat (7½" diameter)	1	●
White Bread	1 slice	●
Whole Wheat Bread*	1 slice	●
Wrap, Low Carb, Wheat, or White	1	●

GRAINS

Food	Amount	
Barley*	⅔ c	●
Bulgur*	1 c	●
Cornmeal	⅔ c	●
Couscous*	½ c	●
Quinoa*	½ c	●
Rice, Brown*	½ c	●
Rice, Chicken	½ c	●
Rice, Dirty	½ c	●
Rice, Fried, Any Type	½ c	●
Rice Pilaf	½ c	●
Rice, Spanish	¾ c	●
Rice, White	½ c	●
Rice, Wild*	⅔ c	●

PASTA AND PIZZA

Food	Amount	
Fettuccine Alfredo	½ c	●
Gnocchi, Cheese, No Sauce	⅓ c	●
Gnocchi, Potato, No Sauce	½ c	●
Gnocchi, Spinach, No Sauce	⅔ c	●
Kugel, Noodle	1 small square	●●
Lasagna, Cheese	⅔ c	●
Lasagna, Meat	⅔ c	●
Lasagna Noodles, No Sauce	1½ noodles	●
Lasagna, Vegetable	¾ c	●
Macaroni and Cheese, Prepared from Box	½ c	●
Macaroni and Cheese, Restaurant or Homemade	½ c	●
Macaroni Salad	½ c	●
Noodles, Egg	⅓ c	●
Noodles, Rice	⅔ c	●

Food	Amount	
Pasta, Cooked	½ c	●
Pasta, Cooked, with Marinara Sauce	⅓ c	●
Pasta, Cooked, Whole Wheat*	⅔ c	●
Pasta, Cooked, Whole Wheat, with Marinara Sauce*	½ c	●
Pasta, Garlic and Oil Sauce	⅔ c	●
Pasta Primavera with Cream Sauce	¾ c	●
Pasta Primavera with Marinara Sauce	½ c	●
Pasta Salad	⅔ c	●
Pasta, Spinach	½ c	●
Pizza, Deep-Dish, One Meat Topping	1 slice	●●
Pizza, Eddie's Pizza	⅓ bar pie	●
Pizza, French Bread	1 piece	●●
Pizza, Kids' Menu, Personal Pizza	½ pie	●
Pizza, Medium Crust, Cheese	1 slice	●●
Pizza, Medium Crust, One Meat Topping	1 slice	●
Pizza Rolls, Tostino's	2 small	●
Pizza, Sicilian Style	1 slice	●
Pizza, Sicilian Style, One Meat Topping	1 slice	●●
Pizza, Single Serving Pie, Cheese	½ pie	●
Pizza, Single Serving Pie, Cheese	1 slice	●
Pizza, Thin Crust, Cheese	1 slice	●●
Pizza, Thin Crust, One Meat Topping	1 slice	●●
Ravioli, Cheese	3	●
Ravioli, Meat	2	●

Shells, Stuffed with Cheese, No Sauce	1½	●
Spaghetti Bolognese	¾ c	●
Spaghetti Carbonara	¾ c	●
Spaghetti, Regular	½ c	●
Spaghetti, Whole Wheat*	⅔ c	●
Spaghetti with Meat Sauce	½ c	●
Tortellini, Beef, No Sauce	7	●
Tortellini, Cheese, No Sauce	7	●
Ziti, Baked, with Meat	½ c	●
Ziti, Baked, without Meat	⅔ c	●
POTATOES		
French Fries, Frozen, Baked without Fat*	10	●
French Fries, Restaurant	8	●
Hash Browns	½ c	●●
Home Fries	½ c	●
Knish, Kasha	1	●
Knish, Potato	½	●
Kugel, Potato	1 small square	●●
Latkes, Potato	1 medium	●
Pierogies, Cheese, Meat, or Potato	1	●
Potato, Baked (2½"–3" diameter)*	⅔	●
Potato, Baked (3½"–4" diameter)*	⅔	●
Potato, Baked*	4 oz	●
Potato, Baked, with Cheese Sauce	⅔	●
Potato, Baked, with Sour Cream and Chives	¾	●
Potatoes, au Gratin	⅔ c	●
Potatoes, Boiled*	⅔ c	●
Potatoes, Garlic Mashed	½ c	●

Potatoes, Mashed, with Fat-Free Milk*	⅔ c	●
Potatoes, Mashed, with Fat-Free Milk and Butter	½ c	●
Potatoes, Mashed, with Whole Milk	1 c	●
Potatoes, Mashed, with Whole Milk and Butter	¾ c	●
Potatoes O'Brien	⅔ c	●
Potato Pancakes, Medium (3½" diameter)	1	●
Potato Pancakes, Small (2½" diameter)	1½	●
Potatoes, Red, White, Bliss, or New*	2 small	●
Potatoes, Scalloped	¾ c	●
Potato Salad	⅔ c	●
Potato Skins with Cheese, Bacon, and Sour Cream	2	●
Potatoes, Tater Tots	5	●
Sweet Potato, Baked (2" diameter, 5" long)*	1	●
Sweet Potato, Baked*	4 oz	●
Sweet Potato, Candied	½ c	●
Sweet Potato Pie	1 slice	●
FRUITS		
Most Fruits, Dried	⅓ c	●
Most Fruits, Fresh*	Unlimited	Free
Ambrosia	⅓ c	●
Applesauce, Sweetened	½ c	●
Applesauce, Unsweetened*	¾ c	●
Canned, in Heavy Syrup	⅔ c	●
Canned, in Light Syrup	1 c	●
Canned, in Water*	1½ c	●
Craisins	¼ c	●
Olives	20	●
Raisins	¼ c	●

Item	Serving	
Raisins, Minibox	2	●
Raisins, Small Box	1	●

VEGETABLES

Item	Serving	
Most Vegetables, Fresh*	Unlimited	Free
Artichoke Hearts	6	●
Artichoke Hearts, Marinated	3	●
Artichoke, Stuffed	½	●
Avocado*	⅓ c sliced (2 oz)	●
Cole Slaw	¼ c	●
Corn, Cream-Style	1 c	●
Corn, Kernels*	¾ c	●
Corn on the Cob*	1	●
Eggplant, Breaded and Fried	3 slices	●
Eggplant Parmigiana, with Sauce	⅔ piece	●
Mushrooms, Marinated	⅓ c	●
Onion Rings, Fried	6	●
Pickles*	Unlimited	Free
Red Peppers, Roasted	½ c	●
Salad, Caesar, with Dressing	2 c	●
Salad, Chef's, without Dressing	3 c	●
Salad Niçoise, without Dressing*	2 c	●
Spinach, Creamed, Frozen	½ c	●
Spinach, Creamed, Restaurant	½ c	●
Stir-Fried Vegetables*	⅔ c	●
Tzimmes	1 small serving	●

BEANS

Item	Serving	
Beans, Baked, Vegetarian, Canned*	½ c	●
Beans, Baked with Pork, Canned	½ c	●
Beans, Most Types, Not Canned, Cooked*	½ c	●
Beans, Refried, Canned	½ c	●
Beans, Refried, Not Canned	⅔ c	●
Chickpeas*	2 Tbsp	●
Edamame, with Pods*	Unlimited	Free
Soybeans*	⅓ c	●
Three Bean Salad, Canned	½ c	●
Three Bean Salad, Not Canned*	½ c	●

NUTS

Item	Serving	
Almonds*	12	●
Brazil Nuts*	6	●
Cashews*	7	●
Chestnuts*	1 oz (3 kernels)	●
Hazelnuts*	10	●
Macadamia Nuts*	5	●
Mixed, Dry-Roasted*	2 Tbsp	●
Peanut Butter, Regular or Reduced-Fat*	1 Tbsp	●
Peanuts*	20	●
Pecans*	6 halves	●
Pine Nuts*	1 Tbsp	●
Pistachios*	20 (2 Tbsp)	●
Pumpkin Seeds, without Shells*	2 Tbsp	●
Sunflower Seeds, with Shells*	⅓ c	●
Sunflower Seeds, without Shells*	2 Tbsp	●
Trail Mix, +/- Chocolate*	2 Tbsp	●
Walnuts*	6 halves	●

SOUPS

Item	Serving	
Borscht, Manischewitz, Low-Calorie*	3 c	●
Borscht, Regular	1 c	●
Broth, Any Type*	Unlimited	Free
Chicken Noodle Soup, Canned, Condensed*	¾ c	●

Food	Serving	
Chicken Noodle Soup, Canned, Ready-To-Serve*	1 c	●
Chicken Noodle Soup, Home-Style*	¾ c	●
Chicken Soup, No Noodles*	Unlimited	Free
Italian Wedding Soup, Canned	⅔ c	●
Italian Wedding Soup, Home-Style	½ c	●
Lentil Soup*	⅔ c	●
Manhattan Clam Chowder, Canned*	1½ c	●
Manhattan Clam Chowder, Home-Style*	¾ c	●
Matzo Ball Soup	1 medium ball	●
Minestrone, Canned*	1 c	●
Minestrone, Home-Style*	½ c	●
Mushroom Soup, Cream of, Home-Style	⅔ c	●
Mushroom Soup, Cream of, Made with Fat-Free Milk*	⅔ c	●
Mushroom Soup, Cream of, Made with Whole Milk	½ c	●
New England Clam Chowder, Home-Style	⅔ c	●
New England Clam Chowder, Canned, Made with Fat-Free Milk*	⅔ c	●
New England Clam Chowder, Canned, Made with Whole Milk	½ c	●
Onion Soup, French-Style, au Gratin	⅔ c	●
Onion Soup, French-Style, au Gratin, 1 Crock	1⅓ c (10 oz)	●
Pea Soup*	⅔ c	●
Ramen Noodle Soup, Any Flavor	1 container	●
Tomato Soup, Canned, Made with Fat-Free Milk*	1 c	●
Tomato Soup, Canned, Made with Water*	1 c	●
Tomato Soup, Canned, Made with Whole Milk	⅔ c	●
Tomato Soup, Cream of	½ c	●
Tomato Soup, Home-Style*	1 c	●
Vegetable Soup*	1 c	●

DIPS, CONDIMENTS, SPREADS, SAUCES, DRESSINGS, OILS		
Alfredo Sauce	⅓ c	●
Artichoke Dip, Baked	3 Tbsp	●
Barbecue Sauce	⅓ c	●
Black Bean Dip, Fat-Free*	½ c	●
Black Bean Sauce	⅓ c	●
Cheddar Cheese Sauce	¼ c	●
Cocktail Sauce	Unlimited	Free
Cranberry Sauce	¼ c	●
Duck Sauce	2 Tbsp	●
Gravy, au Jus, Canned	Unlimited	Free
Gravy, Beef, Brown, Chicken, or Mushroom	⅔ c	●
Gravy, Cream	2 Tbsp	●
Guacamole*	¼ c	●
Hoisin Sauce	3 Tbsp	●
Hollandaise Sauce	¼ c	●
Honey	1½ Tbsp	●
Honey Mustard	¼ c	●
Horseradish	Unlimited	Free
Hot Sauce	Unlimited	Free
Hummus*	¼ c	●
Jelly, Regular	2 Tbsp	●
Jelly, Sugar-Free	Unlimited	Free
Ketchup	Unlimited	Free
Marinara Sauce	½ c	●
Mayonnaise, Canola Oil, Cholesterol-Free	2 Tbsp	●
Mayonnaise, Fat-Free	Unlimited	Free
Mayonnaise, Light	1½ Tbsp	●

Mayonnaise, Low-Fat	4 Tbsp	●
Mayonnaise, Olive Oil	2 Tbsp	●
Mayonnaise, Regular	1½ Tbsp	●
Mustard*	Unlimited	Free
Oil, Any Type	1½ Tbsp	●
Onion Dip	2 Tbsp	●
Pasta Sauce, Jarred, Light	1 c	●
Pasta Sauce, Jarred, Regular	½ c	●
Pesto Sauce	¼ c	●
Salad Dressing, Fat-Free, Italian*	Unlimited	Free
Salad Dressing, Fat-Free, Other Types*	4 Tbsp	●
Salad Dressing, Ginger	2 Tbsp	●
Salad Dressing, Light	2 Tbsp	●
Salad Dressing, Regular	1 Tbsp	●
Salad Dressing, Spray*	Unlimited	Free
Salsa*	Unlimited	Free
Salsa Con Queso	2 Tbsp	●
Soy Sauce	Unlimited	Free
Spinach Dip	3 Tbsp	●
Sugar	2 Tbsp	●
Sugar Packets	4	●
Tartar Sauce	2 Tbsp	●
Teriyaki Sauce	Unlimited	Free
Teriyaki Sauce Marinade	¼ c	●
Tomato Sauce, Canned*	Unlimited	Free

SNACKS

BARS AND TREATS

All-Bran Bar*	1	●
Cereal Bars, Fat-Free	1	●
Cereal Bars, Regular	1	●

Clif Bar	1	●●
Fiber One Bar*	1	●
Fig Bars	2	●
Fruit Roll-Up	1	●
Fruit Snacks	12 pieces	●
Granola Bar, Chocolate-Coated	1	●
Granola Bar, Reduced-Calorie*	1	●
Granola Bar, Regular, Hard	1	●
Granola Bar, Regular, Soft*	1	●
Kashi GoLean Chewy Bar	1	●●
Kashi GoLean Crunchy! Bar*	1	●
Kashi GoLean Roll! Bar*	1	●
Kashi TLC Chewy Bar*	1	●
Kashi TLC Crunchy Bar*	1	●
Luna Bar*	1	●
Nature Valley Granola Bar	1 (½ package)	●
Nutri-Grain, All Types	1	●
PowerBar	1	●
Quaker Granola Bar, Chewy, Regular or Low-Fat	1	●
Rice Krispies Treat	2" square	●

CHIPS, POPCORN, PRETZELS

Bagel Chips, Stacy's, Any Type	10	●
Cheese Puffs, Crunchy, Baked	25	●
Cheese Puffs, Crunchy, Regular	10	●
Cheese Puffs, Puffed	15	●
Corn Chips	15	●
Cracker Jacks	⅓ c	●
Doritos, Baked	15	●

Doritos, Regular	8	●
Pirate's Booty	1½ c	●
Pita Chips, Stacy's, Flavored, Any Type	8	●
Pita Chips, Stacy's, Simply Naked	11	●
Popcorn, Air-Popped*	3 c	●
Popcorn, Caramel	1½ c	●
Popcorn, Cheese-Flavored	3 c	●
Popcorn, Light, Butter	3 c	●
Popcorn, Light, Caramel	2 c	●
Popcorn, Light, Cheese	2 c	●
Popcorn, Light, Plain	3 c	●
Popcorn, Microwave	2 c	●
Popcorn, Microwave, 94% Fat-Free*	3 c	●
Popcorn, Movie Theater, No Butter	3 c	●
Popcorn, Movie Theater, with Butter	2 c	●
Popcorn, Oil-Popped	3 c	●
Popcorn, Store-Bought	1½ c	●
Potato Chips, Baked	10	●
Potato Chips, Light	9	●
Potato Chips, Regular	6	●
Potato Sticks	½ c	●
Pretzels, Bavarian	1	●
Pretzels, Honey, Braided Twists	7	●
Pretzels, Honey-Mustard Pretzel Chips	18	●
Pretzels, Mall Stand (e.g., Auntie Anne's), Butter	1	●
Pretzels, Mall Stand, Cinnamon Sugar	1	●
Pretzels, Mall Stand, No Butter	1	●●

Pretzel, Soft	1	●●
Pretzels, Rods	2	●
Pretzels, Sticks	35 small	●
Pretzels, Twists	20 small	●
Pretzels, Yogurt-Covered	5	●
Rice Cakes, Flavored	2 regular	●
Rice Cakes, Mini, Flavored or Plain	10	●
Rice Cakes, Plain	3 regular	●
Smartfood	1 c	●
Smartfood, Reduced-Fat	2 c	●
Soy Crisps, Stacy's, Any Type	14	●
SunChips	11	●
Tortilla Chips, Baked	12	●
Tortilla Chips, Light	12	●
Tortilla Chips, Regular	8	●
COOKIES		
100-Calorie Pack, Any Type	1	●
Biscotti, Regular Size	1	●
Biscotti, Small Size	1	●
Butter Cookies	2 small	●
Chips Ahoy! Cookies, Mini	3	●
Chips Ahoy! Cookies, Reduced-Fat	2	●
Chips Ahoy! Cookies, Regular	1	●
Chocolate Chip Cookies, Commercially Made (2" diameter)	2	●
Chocolate Chip Cookies, Commercially Made (3½" diameter)	1	●
Chocolate Chip Cookies, Commercially Made, Bite-Size	9	●
Chocolate Chip Cookies, Homemade	1 small	●
Coconut Macaroons	2	●

Cookies, Pepperidge Farm, Any Type	1 large	●
Fortune Cookies	3	●
Fudge Cookies	2	●
Gingerbread Cookies	1	●
Graham Cracker, Crumbs	¼ c	●
Graham Crackers, Chocolate-Covered (2½" square)	1	●
Graham Crackers, Chocolate-Flavored	1 full	●
Graham Crackers, Regular or Reduced-Fat	1 full	●
Macaroons (small)	1	●
Macaroons (large)	1	●
Mallomars	1	●
Mrs. Fields Cookies, Bite-Size	3	●
Mrs. Fields Cookie, Large	1	●
Oatmeal Cookies	1	●
Oreo Cookies, Double Stuf	1	●
Oreo Cookies, Mini	6	●
Oreo Cookies, Reduced-Fat	1	●
Oreo Cookies, Regular	1	●
Peanut Butter Cookies, Commercially Made	1	●
Peanut Butter Cookies, Homemade (3" diameter)	1	●
Shortbread Cookies (2" diameter)	1	●
SnackWells, Cream Sandwich	1	●
SnackWells, Fat-Free, Devil's Food	1	●
Sugar Cookies (3" diameter)	1	●
Sugar Wafer Cookies with Cream (3½" long)	2	●
Vanilla Sandwich Cookies with Cream Filling, Oval	1	●
Vanilla Sandwich Cookies with Cream Filling, Round	2	●
Vanilla Wafer	2	●

CRACKERS		
100-Calorie Pack, Any Type	1	●
Animal Crackers	9	●
Arrowroot Biscuits	5	●
Breadsticks	2	●
Cheese Crackers, Bite-Size	16	●
Cheese Crackers, Peanut Butter Sandwich	5	●
Club Crackers	5	●
Club Crackers, Reduced-Fat	7	●
Crackers with Cheese Filling, Sandwich	4	●
Goldfish Crackers, Regular or Pretzel	40	●
Matzo	¾ board	●
Melba Toast	8 pieces	●
Milk Crackers	2	●
Oyster Crackers	20	●
Ritz Crackers	8	●
Ritz Crisps	16	●
Sabra Hummus with Pretzel Chips	1 container	●●
Saltines, Fat-Free or Regular	6	●
Triscuits, Reduced-Fat	6	●
Triscuits, Regular	5	●
Wasa Crispbread*	3	●
Wheat Thins	10	●
PUDDINGS AND JELL-O		
Corn Pudding	¾ c	●
Jell-O, Flavored, Fat-Free	½ c	●
Jell-O, Flavored, Regular	½ c	●
Jell-O, Flavored, Sugar-Free	Unlimited	Free
Pudding, Any Flavor, Fat-Free, Sugar-Free	⅔ c	●

Food	Amount
Pudding, Ready-to-Eat, Small Containers	1
Pudding, Regular, Made with Any Milk	⅔ c
Rice Pudding, Kozy Shack	½ c
Rice Pudding, Kozy Shack, No Sugar Added	½ c
Rice Pudding, Made with 2% Milk	½ c
Rice Pudding, Made with Whole Milk	½ c
Tapioca Pudding, Made with 2% Milk	½ c
Tapioca Pudding, Made with Whole Milk	½ c
Tapioca Pudding, Ready-to-Eat, Small Container	1

DESSERTS

CAKES, BROWNIES, DOUGHNUTS

Food	Amount
Angel Food	1 slice
Brownie, Fat-Free (2½" square)	1
Brownie, Low-Fat (3" square)	1
Brownie, Regular (2½" square)	1
Cake, with Icing, Homemade or Bakery	1 slice
Cake, with Icing, Store-Bought	1 slice
Carrot Cake with Cream Cheese Frosting	½ slice
Cheesecake, New York–Style	1 slice
Churro	1
Coffee Cake, with Crumb Topping	1 slice
Coffee Cake, Drake's	1½ small
Cupcakes, with Frosting, Bakery	1
Cupcakes, with Frosting, Low-Fat	1 cupcake (1½ oz)

Food	Amount
Cupcakes, Crumbs Bake Shop	1 cupcake
Cupcakes, Hostess, Light	1 cupcake
Cupcakes, Hostess, Regular	1 cupcake
Cupcakes, Magnolia Bakery	1 cupcake
Cupcakes, with Frosting, Store-Bought	1 cupcake
Doughnut	1
Doughnut Holes	3
Doughnut, Mini	1
Frosting	1 Tbsp
Fruit Cake	1 slice
Honey Cake	1 slice
Hostess Cupcakes	1 cupcake
Hostess Ding Dongs	1 cake
Hostess Donettes	1 donette
Hostess Donuts, Glazed	1 doughnut
Hostess Fruit Pie	1
Hostess Ho Hos	3
Hostess Honey Bun, Frosted	1
Hostess Honey Bun, Glazed	1
Hostess Suzy Qs	1 Suzy Q
Hostess Twinkies	1 Twinkie
Pineapple Upside-Down Cake	1 slice
Pound Cake, Bakery, Café, Homemade	1 slice

Pound Cake, Supermarket	1 slice	
Rum Cake	1 slice	
Zwetschkenknödel (Plum Dumpling)	1	

CANDY		
Apple, Candied	1 large	
Butterscotch Candies	5	
Candy Corn	15	
Caramels	5	
Caramels, Chocolate-Covered	3	
Carob	1 oz	
Cherries, Chocolate-Covered	2	
Chocolate, Any Type	1 oz	
Chocolate, Baking, Unsweetened	1 square	
Chocolate Bars, Bites, Most Types	8 pieces	
Chocolate Bars, Fun-Size	1	
Chocolate Bars, Most Types	1	
Chocolate Chips	1 Tbsp	
Chocolate Chips, Sugar-Free	1 Tbsp	
Chocolate, Sugar-Free	1½ oz	
Cotton Candy	1 large serving (1 oz)	
FruitaBü	1 piece	
Fudge, with or without Nuts (2" x 2")	1	
Gummy Bears	12	
Gummy Worms	4	
Hard Candies	4	
Hershey's Kisses, Any Type	4	

Jelly Beans	10	
Licorice	2 ropes	
Lollipops, Large	1	
Lollipops, Small	5	
M&Ms	2 Tbsp	
Marshmallows	4	
Peanuts, Chocolate-Covered	2 Tbsp	
Peeps	3	
Peppermint Hard Candy	4	
Pretzels, Chocolate-Covered	2	
Raisins, Chocolate-Covered	¼ c	
Reese's Pieces	2 Tbsp	
Rolos	3 pieces	
Toblerone, Mini	3 pieces	
Toblerone, Regular	⅓ bar	
Tootsie Rolls	4 pieces	

ICE CREAM AND TOPPINGS		
Bar, Ice Cream, Chocolate-Covered	1	
Bar, Ice Cream, Dove	1	
Butterscotch Topping	2 Tbsp	
Cake, Ice Cream	1 slice	
Caramel Topping	2 Tbsp	
Chipwich	1	
Cone, Cake or Wafer	1	
Cone, Waffle, Large	1	
Frozen Yogurt, Ben & Jerry's, Low-Fat	½ c	
Frozen Yogurt, Fat-Free, No Sugar Added	½ c	

Food	Serving	
Frozen Yogurt, Fat-Free, Sweetened with Sugar	½ c	●
Frozen Yogurt, Häagen-Dazs	½ c	●
Frozen Yogurt, Low-Fat	⅓ c	●
Frozen Yogurt, Regular	¾ c	●
Frozen Yogurt, Yogurt & Such, Fat-Free	1 mini	●
Frozen Yogurt, Yogurt & Such, Low-Fat	1 mini	●
Fudgsicle	1	●
Fudgsicle, Sugar-Free	2	●
Good Humor Ice Cream Bar, Candy Center Crunch	1	●
Good Humor Ice Cream Bar, Chocolate Eclair	1	●●
Good Humor Ice Cream Bar, Cookies & Cream, Light	1	●
Good Humor Ice Cream Bar, Cookies & Cream	1	●
Good Humor Ice Cream Bar, Heath	1	●●
Good Humor Ice Cream Bar, Orange Creamsicle	1	●
Good Humor Ice Cream Bar, Oreo	1	●●
Good Humor Ice Cream Bar, Reese's	1	●●
Good Humor Ice Cream Bar, Strawberry & Cream, Light	1	●
Good Humor Ice Cream Bar, Strawberry Shortcake	1	●●
Good Humor Ice Cream Bar, Toasted Almond	1	●●
Good Humor Ice Cream Bar, Vanilla, Premium	1	●●
Good Humor Ice Cream Cone, King, Giant	1	●●
Good Humor Ice Cream Cone, King, Regular	1	●●
Good Humor Ice Cream Cone, Sundae	1	●●
Good Humor Ice Cream Cup, Any Flavor	½ c	●
Good Humor Ice Cream Sandwich, Chocolate Chip Cookie	1	●●
Good Humor Ice Cream Sandwich, Giant Vanilla	1	●●
Good Humor Ice Cream Sandwich, Low-Fat Vanilla	1	●
Good Humor Ice Cream Sandwich, Vanilla	1	●
Good Humor Snack Pops, Vanilla and Chocolate	1	●●
Hot Fudge	3 Tbsp	●
Hot Fudge, Fat-Free	¼ c	●
Ice Cream, Fat-Free	½ c	●
Ice Cream, Fried	⅓ c	●
Ice Cream, Light	¾ c	●
Ice Cream, Light, Sugar-Free	½ c	●
Ice Cream, Premium	¾ c	●
Ice Cream, Regular	½ c	●
Ice Pops, Frozen, Fruit-Flavored, Regular	2	●
Ice Pops, Frozen, Fruit-Flavored, Sugar-Free	Unlimited	Free
Ices, Ralph's, Cream-Based	½ small (1 scoop)	●
Ices, Ralph's, Noncream	½ small (1 scoop)	●
Ices, Ralph's, No Sugar Added	1 small	●
Milkshake	¾ c (6 oz)	●
Sandwich, Ice Cream	1	●

Item	Portion
Snowcone	⅔ regular
Sorbet, Any Flavor besides Chocolate or Coconut	½ c
Sorbet, Chocolate or Coconut	½ c
Sorbet, Häagen Dazs, Any Flavor	½ c
Sprinkles	1 Tbsp
Syrup, Chocolate	2 Tbsp
Tortoni, Restaurant-Style	1 serving
Whipped Cream, Aerosol, Extra Creamy	⅓ c
Whipped Cream, Aerosol, Fat-Free	Unlimited — Free
Whipped Cream, Aerosol, Light	½ c
Whipped Cream, Aerosol, Original or Chocolate	½ c
Whipped Cream, Cool Whip	⅓ c
Whipped Cream, Cool Whip, Fat-Free	½ c
Whipped Cream, Cool Whip, Light or Sugar-Free	½ c

PIE

Item	Portion
Apple or Other Fruit Pie, Commercially Made (9" diameter)	⅛ pie
Apple or Other Fruit Pie, Homemade or Bakery (9" diameter)	⅛ pie
Apple or Other Fruit Pie, Two Crust (9" diameter)	⅛ pie
Boston Cream Pie (9" diameter)	⅛ pie
Chocolate Mousse Pie, from Mix (9" diameter)	⅛ pie
Cobbler, Fruit	½ c
Coconut Custard (9" diameter)	⅛ pie
Cream Pie, with or without Fruit (9" diameter)	⅛ pie
Pecan Pie (8" diameter)	⅙ pie

Item	Portion
Pie Crust, Graham or Oreo (8" diameter)	⅛ pie
Pie Crust, Regular (8" diameter)	⅛ pie
Pumpkin Pie (8" diameter)	⅙ pie

DRINKS

Item	Portion
Apple Cider	6 fl oz
Apple Juice	6 fl oz
Capri Sun	1 pouch
Cocoa, Homemade or Store-Bought	5 fl oz
Cocoa, Instant, Fat-Free or Sugar-Free	1 packet
Cocoa, Instant, Regular	1 packet
Cranberry Juice Cocktail, Low-Calorie	12 fl oz
Cranberry Juice Cocktail, Regular	6 fl oz
Crystal Light, Any Flavor	Unlimited — Free
Fruit Punch	6 fl oz
Fuze Drink, Regular, Any Flavor	8 fl oz
Fuze Drink, Slenderize, Any Flavor	Unlimited — Free
Gatorade	12 fl oz
Grape Juice	6 fl oz
G2	16 fl oz
Lemonade	8 fl oz
Orange Juice	8 fl oz
Seltzer*	Unlimited — Free
Soda, Diet	Unlimited — Free
Soda, Regular	12 fl oz (1 can)
Tomato Juice	Unlimited — Free
VitaminWater	16 fl oz
VitaminWater10	Unlimited — Free
Yoo-Hoo, Light	12 fl oz

Yoo-Hoo, Regular	6 fl oz	●
Yoo-Hoo, Regular, Box	1 box	●

ETHNIC FOODS

CHINESE FOOD

Black Bean Sauce	⅓ c	●
Brown Sauce	½ c	●
Chow Fun	½ c	●
Chow Mein	½ c	●
Dumplings, Chicken or Shrimp	2	●
Dumplings, Meat	3	●
Dumplings, Vegetarian	3	●
Egg Drop Soup*	1 c	●
Egg Foo Yung, without Gravy	½ serving	●
Egg Rolls, Chicken or Shrimp	1	●
Egg Rolls, Meat	1	●●
Fortune Cookies	3	●
Fried Rice, Any Type	½ c	●
General Tso's Chicken	½ c	●
Gyoza	2	●
Hot-and-Sour Soup	1 c	●
Kung Pao, Any Type	½ c	●
Lo Mein, Any Type	⅔ c	●
Moo Goo Gai Pan	⅔ c	●
Moo Shoo Chicken or Pork, with One Pancake	⅔ c	●
Noodles, Fried	⅔ c	●
Orange Beef	¾ c	●
Orange Chicken	⅔ c	●
Pepper Steak	¾ c	●
Rice, Steamed, Brown* or White	½ c	●

Roast Pork	½ c	●
Sesame Chicken	½ c	●
Sesame Noodles	½ c	●
Shrimp Toast	⅔ piece	●
Soup, Egg Drop	1 c	●
Soup, Wonton, Free Broth	2 wontons	●
Spareribs, Chinese	1 rib	●
Spring Roll	1	●
Sweet-and-Sour Beef or Pork	⅔ c	●
Sweet-and-Sour Chicken or Shrimp	⅔ c	●
Vegetables with Beef	½ c	●
Vegetables with Beef, Steamed*	⅔ c	●
Vegetables with Chicken	½ c	●
Vegetables with Chicken, Steamed*	1 c	●
Vegetables with Pork	⅔ c	●
Vegetables with Pork, Steamed*	⅔ c	●
Vegetables with Shrimp or Tofu	⅔ c	●
Vegetables with Shrimp or Tofu, Steamed*	1½ c	●
Wontons, Fried	1	●
Wontons, Steamed	2	●

JAPANESE FOOD

Edamame, with Pods*	Unlimited	Free
Ginger Salad Dressing	2 Tbsp	●
Gyoza	2	●
Hibachi Chicken	½ c	●
Hibachi Shrimp	½ c	●
Hibachi Steak	½ c	●
Hibachi Vegetables	½ c	●
Katsu, Ahi, Chicken, or Pork	2 slices	●●

Food	Portion	
Maki, Hand Roll, Any Type, with Avocado	1 roll (6 pieces)	●
Maki, Hand Roll, Any Type, without Avocado	1 roll (6 pieces)	●
Maki, Sushi Roll, Any Type, Spicy	4 pieces	●
Maki, Sushi Roll, Any Type, with Avocado	4 pieces	●
Maki, Sushi Roll, Any Type, without Avocado	1 roll (6 pieces)	●
Maki, Sushi Roll, Dragon	4 pieces	●
Maki, Sushi Roll, Philadelphia	4 pieces	●
Maki, Sushi Roll, Shrimp Tempura	4 pieces	●
Maki, Sushi Roll, Spider	4 pieces	●
Miso Soup	1 c	●
Nigiri (Fish Slices on Rice)	2 pieces	●
Ponzu Sauce	Unlimited	Free
Sashimi (Fish without Rice)*	3 pieces	●
Seaweed Salad*	2 oz	●
Shumai	3	●
Soba Noodles	1 c	●
Sukiyaki	1 c	●
Tempura, Shrimp	2	●●
Tempura, Vegetable	½ c	●
Teriyaki, Beef or Chicken	2 slices	●●
Teriyaki, Salmon	6 oz	●●
Teriyaki Sauce	Unlimited	Free
Yakitori	1 skewer	●
MEXICAN FOOD		
Arroz con Pollo	⅔ c	●
Beans, Black*	½ c	●
Beans, Refried	⅔ c	●

Food	Portion	
Black Bean Soup*	⅔ c	●
Burritos, Any Type, Large	½	●●
Burritos, Any Type, Small	1	●●
Carnitas	½ c	●
Chili con Carne	½ c	●
Chuleta	1	●●
Corn Bread, Mexican	1 piece	●●
Dip, Seven-Layer	⅓ c	●
Enchiladas, Any Type	1	●●
Fajitas, Chicken, No Sour Cream or Guacamole	1	●●
Fajitas, Meat, No Sour Cream or Guacamole	1	●●
Fajitas, Vegetable, No Sour Cream or Guacamole	1	●
Guacamole*	¼ c	●
Nachos, Cheese	2	●
Nachos, Cheese and Beef	3	●
Quesadillas, Any Type	½	●
Salsa	Unlimited	Free
Tacos, Any Type	1	●
Taco Salad (no shell)	1 c	●
Taco Shells	1	●
Tamale	½	●
Taquitos, Beef	1	●
Taquitos, Beef and Cheese	1	●
Taquitos, Chicken	2	●
Taquitos, Chicken and Cheese	1	●
Tortilla Chips	8	●

Food	Amount
Tortillas, Flour (8" diameter)	1½
Tostada, Beef	1
Tostada, Chicken	½
MIDDLE EASTERN FOOD	
Baba Ghannouj	¼ c
Falafel	1 small
Falafel Patties	1
Gyro	½
Hummus*	¼ c
Shawarma, Chicken	⅔ c
Shawarma, Chicken	1 thigh
Shish Kebab	1 large skewer
Souvlaki, Chicken	1 skewer
Souvlaki, Chicken, in Pita	1
Souvlaki, Lamb	1 skewer
Souvlaki, Lamb in Pita	1
Tabbouleh	¼ c
Tahini	1 Tbsp
Tzatziki Sauce	2 Tbsp
FAST FOOD	
BURGER KING	
Angus Steak Burger	1
Applesauce, Strawberry-Flavored	1 container
Bacon Double Cheeseburger	1
Biscuit, Bacon, Egg, and Cheese	1
Biscuit, Ham, Egg, and Cheese	1
Biscuit, Sausage, Egg, and Cheese	1

Food	Amount
BK Double Stacker	1
Cheeseburger, Small	1
Cheesy Tots	4 pieces
Chicken Fries	5
Chicken Sandwich, Original	1
Chicken Sandwich, Original, without Mayonnaise	1
Chicken Sandwich, TenderCrisp	1
Chicken Sandwich, TenderGrill	1
Chicken Sandwich, TenderGrill, without Mayonnaise	1
Chicken Tenders	5
Croissan'wich, Bacon, Egg, and Cheese	1
Croissan'wich, Egg and Cheese	1
Croissan'wich, Sausage, Egg, and Cheese	1
Dipping Sauce, BBQ/Sweet-and-Sour	2 packets
Dipping Sauce, Honey Mustard	1 packet
Dipping Sauce, Ranch	⅔ packet
Fish Sandwich	1
Fish Sandwich, without Tartar Sauce	1
French Fries, Large	1 serving
French Fries, Medium	1 serving

Item	Amount	
French Fries, Small	1 serving	●
French Toast Sticks + 1 Packet of Syrup	3 sticks	●●
Hamburger, Small	1	●●
Hash Browns, Large	1 order	●●
Hash Browns, Medium	1 order	●
Hash Browns, Small	1 order	●●
Hershey's Sundae Pie	1	●●
Onion Ring Dipping Sauce	⅔ packet	●
Onion Rings, Large	1 order	●
Onion Rings, Medium	1 order	●●
Onion Rings, Small	1 order	●
Salad, Caesar, with ½ Pack Dressing, No Croutons	1	●●
Salad, Chicken Caesar, No Dressing or Croutons	1	●
Salad Dressing, Caesar	1 packet	●
Salad Dressing, Honey Mustard	1 packet	●●
Salad Dressing, Italian, Light	1 packet	●
Salad Dressing, Ranch	1 packet	●
Salad Dressing, Ranch, Fat-Free	1 packet	●
Salad, Side Garden, No Dressing*	Unlimited	Free
Salad, Shrimp Caesar, No Dressing or Croutons*	1	●
Salad, TenderCrisp Chicken, without Dressing	1	●
Salad, TenderGrill Chicken, without Dressing*	1	●
Shake, Chocolate or Vanilla	1 small	●

Item	Amount	
Shake, Oreo Sundae	1 small	●●
Veggie Burger with Mayo	1	●
Veggie Burger without Mayo*	1	●●
Whopper, No Cheese, No Mayonnaise	1	●●●
Whopper, No Cheese, with Mayonnaise	1	●●●
Whopper, with Cheese, No Mayonnaise	1	●●
Whopper, with Cheese, with Mayonnaise	1	●●
Whopper Jr., No Mayonnaise, No Cheese	1	●●
Whopper Jr., No Mayonnaise, with Cheese	1	●●
Whopper Jr., with Mayonnaise, No Cheese	1	●
Whopper Jr., with Mayonnaise, with Cheese	1	●
KFC		
Apple Pie Minis	2	●
Applesauce	1 serving	●
Baked Beans	1 serving	●
Biscuit	1	●
Cake, Double Chocolate Chip	1 slice	●●
Chicken and Biscuit Bowl	1	●●
Chicken Breast, Extra Crispy	1	●
Chicken Breast, No Skin*	1	●

Food	Servings	Points
Chicken Breast, Original Recipe	1	●
Chicken Drumstick, Either Type	1	●
Chicken Pot Pie	1	●●
Chicken Sandwich, Double Crunch	1	●●●
Chicken Sandwich, Honey BBQ	1	●●
Chicken Sandwich, Tender Roast	1	●
Chicken Sandwich, Tender Roast, without Sauce	1	●●
Chicken Thigh, Extra Crispy	1	●
Chicken Thigh, Original Recipe	1	●●
Chicken Wing, Extra Crispy	1	●
Chicken Wing, Original Recipe	1	●
Cole Slaw	1 serving	●
Cookie	2	●●
Corn on the Cob (3")*	1	●
Corn on the Cob (5½")*	1	●
Crispy Strips	2	●
Famous Bowl, Mashed Potatoes and Gravy	1	●●
Famous Bowl, Rice and Gravy	1	●●
Green Beans*	Unlimited	Free
Macaroni and Cheese	1 serving	●
Mashed Potatoes, with or without Gravy	1 serving	●
Popcorn Chicken, Individual Serving	1	●

Food	Servings	Points
Popcorn Chicken, Kid's Serving	1	●●
Popcorn Chicken, Large Serving	1	●●
Potato Salad	1 serving	●
Potato Wedges	1 serving	●●
Rice	1 serving	●
Salad, BLT, Crispy, No Dressing or Croutons	1	●●
Salad, BLT, Roasted, No Dressing or Croutons	1	●
Salad, Caesar, Crispy, No Dressing or Croutons	1	●
Salad, Caesar, Roasted, No Dressing or Croutons	1	●
Salad Dressing, Creamy Caesar or Ranch	1 serving	●
Salad Dressing, Light Italian or Fat-Free Ranch*	Unlimited	Free
Salad Dressing, Other Fat-Free	1	●
Snacker, BBQ	1	●
Snacker, Other Types	1	●●
Sweet Potato Pie	1 slice	●●
Twister, Crispy	1	●●
Twister, Oven Roasted	1	●
Twister, Oven Roasted, without Sauce	1	●●
Wings, Any Type	2	●

MCDONALD'S		
Apple Dippers, with Caramel Sauce	1 serving	●
Apple Dippers, without Caramel Sauce	Unlimited	Free
Apple Pie	1 serving	●●
Bacon, Egg, and Cheese Biscuit	1	●
Big Mac	1	●●
Big N' Tasty	1	●●
Big N' Tasty with Cheese	1	●●
Biscuit	1	●
Cheeseburger	1	●●
Chicken McGrill	1	●
Chicken McGrill, without Mayonnaise	1	●●
Chicken McNuggets	4	●
Chicken Selects	3	●
Cinnamon Roll	1	●
Cookie, Any Type	1	●
Cookies, McDonaldland	1 package	●●
Crispy Chicken Classic Sandwich	1	●●
Crispy Chicken Club Sandwich	1	●●
Crispy Chicken Ranch BLT Sandwich	1	●●

Egg McMuffin	1	●●
English Muffin	1	●
Filet-O-Fish	1	●
French Fries, Large	1	●●
French Fries, Medium	1	●
French Fries, Small	1	●
Fruit 'n Yogurt Parfait	1 serving	●
Grilled Chicken Classic Sandwich	1	●●
Grilled Chicken Club Sandwich	1	●●
Grilled Chicken Ranch BLT Sandwich	1	●●
Hamburger	1	●●
Hash Browns	1 serving	●
Hot Cakes, No Syrup or Margarine	2	●
Hot Cake Syrup	1 packet	●
McChicken	1	●
McFlurry	1	●●
McGriddles, Egg, Cheese, and Bacon	1	●●
McGriddles, Egg, Cheese, and Sausage	1	●●
McRib	1	●
McSkillet Burrito with Sausage or Steak	1	●●●

Item	Amount	
Quarter Pounder with Cheese	1	●●
Quarter Pounder without Cheese	1	●●●
Salad, Crispy Chicken, Any Type, No Dressing	1	●
Salad Dressing, Balsamic Low-Fat*	Unlimited	Free
Salad Dressing, Low-Fat Sesame	1 packet	●
Salad Dressing, Other Types	1 packet	●
Salad, Fruit and Walnut*	1	●●
Salad, Fruit and Walnut, Snack Size*	1	●
Salad, Grilled Chicken, Any Type, No Dressing*	1	●
Salad, No Chicken, Any Type, No Dressing*	Unlimited	Free
Sauce, BBQ, Honey Mustard, or Sweet 'n Sour	2 servings	●
Sauce, Ranch	1 serving	●
Sausage Biscuit	1	●
Sausage Biscuit with Egg	1	●●
Sausage Burrito	1	●●
Sausage McMuffin	1	●
Sausage McMuffin with Egg	1	●●
Sausage Patty	2	●●
Scrambled Eggs	1 serving	●
Shake (12 fl oz), Any Type	1	●●

Item	Amount	
Snack Wrap, Chicken, Crispy, Any Type	1	●
Snack Wrap, Chicken, Grilled, Any Type	1	●●
Sundae, Any Type	1	●●●
Vanilla Reduced-Fat Ice-Cream Cone	1	●

MOE'S SOUTHWEST GRILL

All values imply no queso, sour cream, guacamole, or grilled vegetables. Items may include chicken, ground beef, steak, or tofu.

Item	Amount	
Beans Side Dish (6 oz bowl)	1	●
Mini Masterpiece	1 order	●●
Moo Moo Mr. Cow	1 order	●
Power Wagon, Hard Shell	1 order	●
Power Wagon, Soft Shell	1 order	●
Quesadilla, Instant Friend or Super Kingpin	1	●●
Quesadilla, John Coctostan	½	●
Rice Side Dish (6 oz bowl)	1	●
Soup, Baja Chicken Enchilada (6 oz bowl)	1	●
Taco, Funk Meister, Hard or Soft	1	●●
Taco, Overachiever, Hard or Soft	1	●●
Taco, Unanimous Decision, Hard or Soft	1	●●

PIZZA HUT

Note: Medium Pie = 12"

Item	Amount	
Breadstick, Plain	1	●
Cheese Stick	1	●

Item	Amount
Cinnamon Sticks	2
Cinnamon Sticks Dip Cup, White King	1
Dessert Pizza	1 slice
Fit N' Delicious Pizza, Medium Pie, Any Type	2 slices
Hand Tossed Pizza, Medium Pie, Any but Meat Lover's	1 slice
Hand Tossed Pizza, Medium Pie, Meat Lover's	1 slice
Pan Pizza, Medium Pie, Any but Meat Lover's	1 slice
Pan Pizza, Medium Pie, Meat Lover's	1 slice
Personal Pan Pizza (6"), Any but Meat Lover's	⅓ pie
Personal Pan Pizza (6"), Meat Lover's	⅓ pie
Salad Dressing, Light, Any Type	2 Tbsp
Salad Dressing, Regular, Any Type	1 Tbsp
Thin 'N Crispy, Pizza Medium Pie, Any but Meat Lover's	1 slice
Thin 'N Crispy Pizza, Medium Pie, Meat Lover's	1 slice
Wings	3
Wing Sauce (1½ oz container)	1
SUBWAY	
Bread, Any Type (6")	1 roll
Bread, Mini, Any Type	1 roll
Breakfast Omelet Sandwich, Cheese (6")	1
Breakfast Omelet Sandwich, Cold Cut Combo (6")	1
Breakfast Omelet Sandwich, Ham and Cheese (6")	1

Item	Amount
Breakfast Omelet Sandwich, Steak and Cheese (6")	1
Breakfast Omelet Sandwich, Tuna (6")	1
Cheese, Added to Sandwich	3 small pieces
Chocolate Chip Cookie	1
Mayonnaise, Light	2 Tbsp
Mayonnaise, Regular	1½ Tbsp
Mini Sub, Ham*	1
Mini Sub, Roast Beef*	1
Mini Sub, Tuna	1
Mini Sub, Turkey*	1
Salad, BMT, No Dressing	1
Salad, Chicken or Ham, No Dressing*	1
Salad, Cold Cut Combo, No Dressing	1
Salad Dressing, Fat-Free, Italian*	Unlimited — Free
Salad Dressing, Fat-Free, Other Types	2 Tbsp
Salad Dressing, Regular, Any Type	1 packet
Salad, Mediterranean Chicken, No Dressing*	1
Salad, Subway Club, No Dressing*	1
Salad, Turkey or Turkey and Ham, No Dressing*	1
Salad, Veggie Delite, No Dressing*	Unlimited — Free
Sandwich, Ham*	1
Sandwich, Roast Beef*	1

Sandwich, Turkey Breast*	1	⬤⬤
Sauce, Chipotle, Amount on Wrap or Sandwich	1 order	⬤
Sauce, Dijon Horseradish	1 order	⬤
Sauce, Honey Mustard, Fat-Free	Unlimited	Free
Sauce, Ranch, Amount on Wrap or Sandwich	1 order	⬤
Sauce, Sweet Onion, Fat-Free	Unlimited	Free
Sub, Chicken and Bacon Ranch (6")	1	⬤⬤
Sub, Club (6")	1	⬤⬤
Sub, Ham (6")*	1	⬤⬤
Sub, Ham and Cheese (6")*	1	⬤⬤
Sub, Italian BMT (6")	1	⬤
Sub, Meatball Marinara (6")	1	⬤⬤
Sub, Roast Beef (6")*	1	⬤⬤
Sub, Roasted Chicken Breast (6")*	1	⬤⬤
Sub, Spicy Italian (6")	1	⬤⬤
Sub, Steak and Cheese (6")	1	⬤
Sub, Subway Melt (6")	1	⬤
Sub, Sweet Onion Chicken Teriyaki (6")*	1	⬤⬤
Sub, Turkey or Turkey and Ham (6")*	1	⬤⬤

Sub, Veggie Delite (6")*	1	⬤⬤
Wrap, Chicken Breast	1	⬤
Wrap, Ham	1	⬤
Wrap, No Filling	1	⬤⬤
Wrap, Roast Beef	1	⬤
Wrap, Subway Club	1	⬤
Wrap, Sweet Onion Chicken Teriyaki	1	⬤
Wrap, Turkey	1	⬤
Wrap, Turkey and Ham	1	⬤
Wrap, Veggie	1	⬤
WENDY'S		
Bacon Cheeseburger, Junior	1	⬤⬤
Baked Potato*	1	⬤⬤
Baked Potato with Sour Cream and Chives	1	⬤
Cheeseburger, Junior	1	⬤⬤
Chicken Go Wrap, Any Type	1	⬤⬤
Chicken Nuggets	4	⬤
Chicken Nuggets	8	⬤
Chicken Nugget Sauce, BBQ or Sweet and Sour	2 packets	⬤
Chicken Nugget Sauce, Honey Mustard or Ranch	1 packet	⬤
Chicken Sandwich, Club	1	⬤⬤
Chicken Sandwich, Crispy	1	⬤
Chicken Sandwich, Fillet	1	⬤

Food	Serving
Chicken Sandwich, Grilled, Ultimate	1
Chili, Large	1
Chili, Small	1
French Fries, Kid's Meal Size	1
French Fries, Medium	1
French Fries, Small	1
Frosty, Junior	1
Frosty, Small	1
Hamburger, Junior	1
Hamburger, Single, with Everything	1
Oranges, Mandarin*	Unlimited Free

Salads Do Not Include Dressing

Food	Serving
Salad, Chicken BLT, No Croutons	1
Salad, Chicken BLT, with Croutons	1
Salad, Chicken Caesar, No Croutons	1

Food	Serving
Salad, Chicken Caesar, with Croutons	1
Salad, Mandarin Chicken, No Noodles or Almonds*	1
Salad, Mandarin Chicken, with Noodles and Almonds	1
Salad, Southwest Taco, No Sour Cream or Tortillas	1
Salad, Southwest Taco, with Sour Cream andTortillas	1
Salad Dressing, Blue Cheese	1 order
Salad Dressing, Caesar	1 order
Salad Dressing, Chipotle Ranch	1 order
Salad Dressing, French, Fat-Free	1 order
Salad Dressing, Honey Mustard	1 order
Salad Dressing, Honey Mustard, Low-Fat	1 order
Salad Dressing, Italian Vinaigrette	¾ order
Salad Dressing, Oriental Sesame	1 order
Salad Dressing, Ranch	1 order
Salad Dressing, Ranch, Reduced-Fat	1 order
Salad Dressing, Thousand Island	1 order

Endnotes

● ● ●

Introduction

1. D. S. Freedman, Z. Mei, S. R. Srinivasan, G. S. Berenson, and W. H. Dietz, "Cardiovascular Risk Factors and Excess Adiposity among Overweight Children and Adolescents: The Bogalusa Heart Study," *Journal of Pediatrics* 150, no. 1 (January 2007): 12–17.e2.
2. S. J. Olshansky, D. J. Passaro, R. C. Hershow, J. Layden, B. A. Carnes, J. Brody, L. Hayflick, R. N. Butler, D. B. Allison, and D. S. Ludwig, "A Potential Decline in Life Expectancy in the United States in the 21st Century," *New England Journal of Medicine* 352, no. 11 (March 17, 2005): 1138–45.
3. Susan Okie, *Fed Up!* (Washington, DC: Joseph Henry Press, 2005), 5.

Chapter 2

1. A. M. Albertson, G. H. Anderson, S. J. Crockett, and M. T. Goebel, "Ready-to-Eat Cereal Consumption: Its Relationship with BMI and Nutrient Intake of Children Aged 4 to 12 Years," *Journal of the American Dietetic Association* 103 (2003): 1613–19.

Chapter 4

1. J. Woo, T. Kwok, J. Leung, and N. Tang, "Dietary Intake, Blood Pressure and Osteoporosis," *Journal of Human Hypertension* 23 (2009): 451–55.

Chapter 6

1. D. M. Matheson, J. D. Killen, Y. Wang, A. Varady, and T. N. Robinson, "Children's Food Consumption during Television Viewing," *American Journal of Clinical Nutrition* 79 (2004): 1088–94.
2. D. L. Borzekowski and T. N. Robinson, "The 30-Second Effect: An Experiment Revealing the Impact of Television Commercials on Food Preferences of Preschoolers," *Journal of the American Dietetic Association* 101, no. 1 (January 2001): 42–46.

Chapter 10

1. A. M. Adachi-Mejia, B. A. Primack, M. L. Beach, L. Titus-Ernstoff, M. R. Longacre, J. E. Weiss, M. A. Dalton, "Influence of Movie Smoking Exposure and Team Sports Participation on Established Smoking," *Archives of Pediatric and Adolescent Medicine* 163, no. 7 (2009): 638–43. This study shows that team sports lead to decreased rates of teen smoking.

Chapter 11

1. L. H. Epstein, C. C. Gordy, H. A. Raynor, M. Beddome, C. K. Kilanowski, and R. Paluch, "Increasing Fruit and Vegetable Intake and Decreasing Fat and Sugar Intake in Families at Risk for Childhood Obesity," *Obesity Research* 9, no. 3 (March 2001): 171–78.

Index

Underscored page references indicate sidebars and tables. **Boldface** references indicate photographs and illustrations.